You Just Don't Die!

The Consciousness of Living to 100 and Beyond

STEPHEN LAU

DEDICATION

This book is dedicated to those who believe that tomorrow Is just another day and is always within reach.

CONTENTS

Acknowledgments   i

Introduction   1

ONE   Consciousness Is Everything   5

TWO   Consciousness of Breath   13

THREE   Consciousness of Thinking   27

FOUR   Consciousness of Wellness   37

FIVE   Consciousness of Living   67

SIX   Consciousness of Changes and Challenges   77

SEVEN   Consciousness of Being   107

EIGHT   You Just Don't Die!   117

A   Recipes for Living to 100 and Beyond   127

B   Wisdom of Centenarians   135

C   The Miracle of Meditation   139

C   Bibliography   143

D   About Stephen Lau   145

ACKNOWLEDGMENTS

. The quotes from Lao Tzu's "Tao Te Ching" are taken from the author's own book "The Complete Tao Te Ching in Plain English", and all the Biblical quotes are from New International Version (NIV).

INTRODUCTION

"No one wants to die. Even people who want to go to heaven don't want to die to get there. And yet death is the final destination we all share." **Steve Job**

"As no one has power over the wind to contain it,
  so no one has power over the time of their death.
As no one is discharged in time of war,
  so wickedness will not release those who practice it." (**Ecclesiastes** 8: 8)

Human Existence

We all exist in this world. For the believers, their existence is a result of the Creator's unfathomable plan for them; for the non-believers, their existence comes from their parents. No matter who we are, we don't have much of a choice, except to continue to exist. According to a 2013 report of the Substance Abuse and Mental Health Services

Administration, nearly one in five American adults (43.8 millions) had some form of mental illness. Surprisingly, not too many of those who were depressed would want to commit suicide or end their lives prematurely; they just wanted to continue to live a life maybe that was different from what they were currently living. In other words, irrespective of our mental conditions or current situations, the majority of us would still want to continue to exist in this world—maybe just wishing we could continue living our lives in a happier and more contented way for a little longer.

The Unrealistic Quest

In ancient times, many individuals were in quest of immortality, especially those in power. For example, **Qin Shi Huang (秦始皇)** (259 BC - 210 BC), the First Emperor of China, had made many futile attempts to discover and access legendary sources of immortality during his relatively short lifespan. Another example, the ancient pharaohs of Egypt might not have been on a quest for immortality because they earnestly believed that they were already immortal; nevertheless, they had spent an enormous amount of resources into retarding the decay of their physical bodies, as well as into building spectacular pyramids and grand tombs in which they could preserve their wealth and riches for their immortality.

The Realistic Realities

Nowadays, we all know the reality that all humans are mortal and that death is as inevitable as day becoming night.

"Is there anything we can do about our mortality?" This might be a question that many of us would like to ask ourselves.

First of all, man's perceptions of mortality always change

with age and time. If you ask a young adult if he or she would want to live long, probably the answer is "I don't know" or "I just don't want to grow *too* old and decrepit, like my grand-parents." The young adult's perspective of mortality also explains why many of the younger generation are living a reckless lifestyle as if there is no tomorrow.

Naturally, their perception of mortality would change over the years as they grow older with a family of children, or if they have a successful career with all the trimmings of a luxurious lifestyle that they would like to continue. A longer lifespan would then become an extension of their own legacy or continuation of their enjoyment of the fruits of their own accomplishments. The inscription on the tombstone of **Bruce Lee** (李小龍), the Hollywood actor, reads: "The key to immortality is first living a life worth remembering." That says much about the hope of many to extend beyond the grave.

As aging continues, the fear of death or the unknown might also dawn on humans, driving some of the elderly into craving a longer lifespan in order to delay and defer the inevitable.

Indeed, many people may have different perspectives of their own mortality, depending on their upbringing, the life experiences they have gone though, their religious beliefs, as well as the meanings of death and dying to them. As a result of the differences, some may focus too much on death to the extent of creating death anxiety, while others may deliberately deny the existence of death, just like the ostrich burying its head in the sand.

Since the beginning of the 20th century, the life expectancy of Americans has significantly increased from 47 to almost 80. How long do you wish to live, if you just don't die? And what would you do with your life, if you just don't die?

The objective of this book is neither to convince you to crave longevity, nor to show you how to live to one hundred and beyond. It simply presents you with the consciousness of living the rest of your years as if everything is a miracle—if you just don't die!

Stephen Lau

ONE

CONSCIOUSNESS IS EVERYTHING

"The key to growth is the introduction of higher dimensions of consciousness into our awareness." **Lao Tzu**

What Is Consciousness?

Consciousness is *everything*; if you are not conscious, you are not living your life, if not already dead.

What is consciousness? Being conscious is a "special quality of the mind" that permits us to *know* both that we exist and that the things around us exist too. Surprisingly, some of us may not have this consciousness.

Life is an inner journey that requires consciousness of the body and the mind, together with that of the soul, to continue to make its progress in the right direction in order to reach its final destination. Unfortunately, since the beginning of time, many people have traveled the same journey of life but without reaching their destinations because they simply lack their consciousness of the body, and the mind—not to mention that of the soul—to guide them along that journey.

Consciousness comes from the mind, which is created by the brain. **Hippocrates** (460 - 370 BC), the father of modern medicine, was one of the first scientists to observe and notice that people with brain damage tended to lose their mental abilities. He realized that the mind is created by the brain, and the mind crumbles piece by piece as the brain dies.

The human brain creates the consciousness of the mind, giving humans pleasures and displeasures, happiness and unhappiness, as well as many other positive and negative emotions and thoughts. They become our experiences which are stored in our minds, and these experiences also become our memories that generate our subsequent thoughts—they are the byproducts with which we weave the realities in our lives. Therefore, consciousness is the capability of the mind to see them as they are. Without consciousness, which is knowing what is happening in the mind, you just obediently follow what your mind tells you. That is to say, you have become a slave to your thinking, instead of being the master of your own thoughts.

Consciousness is probing deep into the conscious mind: asking meaningful and relevant questions, and then seeking self-enlightening answers to all the questions asked. After all, throughout one's life journey, one has to ask many different questions at different stages, and seeking different answers from the questions asked. In order to reach the destination of one's life journey. consciousness of the mind is a necessity, and not an option.

Consciousness of the Basics of Life

Be conscious of the basics of mortality: aging, premature aging, and longevity.

Aging

The passage of time is inevitable and eternal. Aging begins as early as from young adulthood (around age 20 to 40) to middle adulthood (around age 40 to 65), and continues to old age (beginning at the age of retirement, approximately at age 65). Aging occurs throughout most of one's lifespan. The aging process is an accumulation of changes, which may be subtle or sudden, and even drastic, that progressively lead to disease, degeneration, and ultimately death. Truly, you cannot die merely of old age; your ultimate demise is caused by advancing age itself, as well as by the diseases and degenerative conditions that accompany it.

Aging is difficult to define, but you will know it when you see it, or experience it firsthand yourself. In brief, aging is a steady decline in health and wellness, instrumental in shortening lifespan; and the aging process is the duration during which such changes occur.

The hard facts of aging

Whether you like it or not, your biological clock is ticking, and this will happen to various systems in your body:

- Your heart will pump less blood, and your arteries will become stiffer and less flexible, resulting in high blood pressure—a common health problem that often increases with age.
- With less oxygen and nutrients from the heart, your lungs will also become less efficient in getting and distributing oxygen to different organs and membranes of your body.

- Your brain size will slowly and gradually reduce by approximately 10 percent between the age of 30 and 70. Loss of short-term memory will become increasingly more acute and evident.
- Your bone mass will reduce, making it more brittle and fragile. Your body size will shrink as you lose your muscle mass.

Your biological clock is continuously ticking, whether you are conscious of it or not. Your mortality has been pre-programmed into your biological organisms and your body cells. Theoretically, you may have an indefinite lifespan through the division, the rejuvenation, and the regeneration of your body cells and organisms—*if* they are still healthy and fully functional. Although your genes may have pre-determined the speed of your biological clock, you can still slow down the speed of aging—*if* you still have good health.

So, what is good health? Is being healthy synonymous with the absence of disease?

According to the United States Public Health Service, good health is "preventing premature death, and preventing disability, preserving a physical environment that supports human life, cultivating family and community support, enhancing each individual's inherent abilities to respond and to act, and assuring that all Americans achieve and maintain a maximum level of functioning." This statement probably sums up what you need to do in order to be younger and healthier for longer; it says *everything* about aging.

Premature aging

The truth of the matter is that you age, just like everyone else does. The point in question is *how* you can delay that aging process in order to make you not only feel but also look younger and healthier for longer—or, at least, not making you age more quickly than you are supposed to.

Unfortunately, many of us have fallen victims to the accelerated aging syndrome, or premature aging.

Accelerated aging syndrome

According to **Steven Masley**, M.D., the former medical director of the Pritikin Longevity Center in St. Petersburg, Florida, you may have the potentials for accelerated aging, if you have just any *three* of the following:

- A fast blood sugar level of more than 100 mg/dl
- A blood pressure higher than 130/85
- A waist larger than 35 inches for women and 40 inches for men
- Good cholesterol level (HDL) less than 40 mg/dl for men, and 50 mg/dl for women
- Triglyceride (a certain type of fat in your blood) levels greater than 150 mg/dl

Factors contributing to premature aging

There are several factors that increase the predisposition to accelerated aging:

- Your diet: you are what you eat, and you become what you eat.
- Your lifestyle: life on the fast lane often leads to faster aging.
- Your physical inactivity: immobility brings about stagnation and degeneration.
- Your stress level: stress kills your brain cells, predisposing you to premature aging.

- Your disease and physical pain: disease and pain have a devastating impact on both the body and the mind

Damaging free radicals

Your body is composed of many different types of cells, made up of many different types of molecules.

Free radicals are molecules that contain *unpaired* electrons. Since electrons have a very strong tendency to co-exist in a paired rather than in an unpaired state, free radicals *indiscriminately* pick up electrons from other healthy molecules close by. This chemical reaction converts those otherwise "healthy" molecules into free radicals, and thus setting up a chain reaction that can cause substantial biological damage to cells. Free radicals are highly reactive, damaging not only cells but also chemicals in your body, such as enzymes (for digestion), making them less effective and efficient.

Aging causes oxidation, which literally means "rusting." Free radicals cause oxidative damage to cells and tissues. Free radicals do not make you younger and healthier for longer; quite the contrary, they age you prematurely and contribute to many diseases, including cancer and heart disease, among others.

Free radicals occur naturally as byproducts of oxidation, such as during respiration and other chemical processes. For example, during your breathing, life-giving oxygen is produced while harmful carbon dioxide is released; digestion is another oxidation process, in which your body obtains its energy from food through oxidation, during which free radicals are also generated in the form of waste buildup. Ironically, what gives life may also take away life indirectly.

Free radicals are normally present in your body in small

numbers, without causing too much harm. However, over the long haul, the accumulation of these free radicals may cause irreparable damage to your body cells and tissues, if such accumulation is unchecked.

In addition, free radicals can also be caused by external factors, such as alcohol, nicotine, chemicals from foods and toxic pharmaceutical drugs, heavy metals, such as cadmium and lead, from the environment, radiation from the sun and other sources.

Longevity

The word "longevity" has its origin from the Latin word "longaevitas", which comes from the word "longus" or long, and "aevu" or age.

Genes do not cause aging but they do indirectly affect longevity in that they may pre-determine the rate of division, rejuvenation, and regeneration of body cells and organisms.

Consciousness of longevity involves your awareness of preventative intervention and detection of early signs of medical conditions that could potentially affect longevity.

Consciousness of Questions and Answers

To live to 100 and beyond—if you just don't die—you must ask questions about life; after all, living is about asking questions and seeking answers to the questions asked, and thereby instrumental in providing wisdom or a blueprint to continue the rest of your life journey.

The first question you should consciously ask yourself is: *How long do you wish to live?* Of course, that is only a hypothetical question because you really don't have much of a choice—unless you would like to purposely end your life prematurely. Naturally, the answer to that question might also change over different phases in your life, depending on the quality of your life in that particular phase.

The second question you should consciously ask yourself is: *Why do you want to live long, or why not?* This question will be naturally followed by the third question: *How do you live long, or what can make you desire to live longer?*

The final question—if you just don't die—is: *How should you live the rest of your life?*

Consciousness Is Everything

Consciousness is, in fact, *everything* in your life and living. Consciousness is your mental awareness of the self, of others, and of the world around you. Without thinking, which is consciousness of the mind, you are not living; you are simply existing.

Albert Einstein once said, "Thinking is difficult; that's why so few people do it." Thinking is a process of self-intuition through asking relevant questions to create self-awareness and self-introspection. It is the natural habit of the human mind to try to solve problems by asking questions. Through solving problems, the mind can then make things *happen*. Asking relevant questions is self-empowerment of human mind to create wisdom because it creates the intent to learn, to discover, and then to change. Without change, life then becomes static, boring, and ultimately unhappy and meaningless.

If You Just Don't Die

It is your own consciousness that makes things *happen* in your life so that you can continue the rest of your life journey and live as if everything is a miracle—even to 100 and beyond, if you just don't die!

TWO

CONSCIOUSNESS OF BREATH

"You have a choice. Live or die. Every breath is a choice. Every minute is a choice. To be or not to be." **Chuck Palahniuk**

Life is made up of many breaths. Therefore, your consciousness of your breath is your consciousness of life, as well as of many other things in life. Consciousness of breath begins with breathing.

Consciousness of the Importance of Breath

Are you constantly conscious of your breath—your breathing in and breathing out? Most people aren't.

Breathing is the most subconscious and yet the most important activity in human life. Unfortunately, many of us aren't conscious of it.

Breath and the Bible

The Bible has made references to the importance of breath from God, which is not only life itself but also divine understanding.

> "And the LORD God formed man *of* the dust of the ground, and breathed into his nostrils the breath of life; and man became a living being." (**Genesis** 2:7)

> "In whose hand *is* the life of every living thing, And the breath of all mankind?" (**Job**: 12:10)

> "But *there is* a spirit in man, And the breath of the Almighty gives him understanding." (**Job** 32:8)

Breath and Chinese medicine

According to Traditional Chinese Medicine (TCM), the two most important health regulators of the human body are *breath* and *blood flow*. Optimum breathing brings oxygen to every cell in your organs and tissues; while smooth blood flow carries nutrients to nourish them. The effective and efficient functioning of breath and blood flow is conducive to the balance and harmony of the *yin* and the *yang*, which are the fundamentals of Chinese medicine.

The Chinese breath is longevity breath because it helps you not only get but also use oxygen 24 hours a day. The Chinese breath lowers your blood pressure, calms your nerves, and alleviates your body pain, if you have any. In addition, the Chinese breath improves the overall emotional health through clarity of thinking, and even detoxifies your body system through internal cleansing. The explanation is that your body organs, including the liver, spleen, kidneys, glands, and digestive valves are all connected to the diaphragm (the muscles between the lungs and the abdomen), which basically moves the air circulation within the body when you breathe in and breathe out. Without moving the diaphragm muscles, and using only the muscles of the chest, you breathe only partially and incompletely. As a strong testament to its significance, the Chinese breath focuses on correct breathing with the diaphragm; Chinese exercises, such as Tai Chi and Qi Gong, also focus on the importance of breath.

The Chinese breath is also related to *qi*, which can be interpreted as the "life energy" or "life force," which flows within the human body. According to TCM theory, *qi* is the "vital substance" constituting the human body; it also refers to the physiological functions of organs and meridians (energy highways assessing different parts of the body and their respective organs). It should be pointed out that breath and *qi* are similar but not quite the same. The air that flows through the lungs at each breath has many similarities to the *qi* energy flowing through the meridians of the body. That goes for oxygen as well; the substance that breathing transports to the blood, and the blood distributes to all of the body—just like *qi* energy traveling through its many meridians.

Consciousness of Correct Breathing

Breathing has to do with the lungs, which serve two main functions: to get life-giving oxygen from the air into the body, and to remove toxic carbon dioxide from the body. Therefore, it is important to be conscious of a longer breathing out than a breathing in so as to maximize the removal of the toxic carbon dioxide from the lungs.

But the functioning of the lungs may have compromised due to aging or incorrect breathing over decades of misuse. Compromised breathing is often due to changes in bones and muscles of the chest and the spine: bones becoming thinner can change the shape of your ribcage, making it less capable of expanding and contracting during your breathing. In addition; the muscles supporting your breathing and your diaphragm may also have weakened due to age, such that you have difficulty in breathing in and breathing out enough air. Furthermore, the lung tissues near your airway may have weakened, leading to their incapability to completely open and close the airways. As a result, air that is trapped in your lungs may also prevent efficient inhaling and exhaling, thus making it harder for you to breathe. On top of these, a weakened immune system may also make your lungs become more vulnerable to infections and less capable of recovering from your exposure to smoke and other toxic environmental particles. To add insult to injury, as you age, your nervous system that controls your breathing may have become less functional, making your airways more sensitive to germs and infections. As you continue to increase in age, your lungs may become more vulnerable to lung infections, such as bronchitis and pneumonia, resulting in many health-related problems due to a lower oxygen level in your blood supply.

First and foremost, learn how to breathe *correctly*; many people don't breathe right because they are not conscious of their breathing. Breathing right may help you in many ways in your everyday life and living. Remember, a healthy mind always has an easy breath, giving a relaxed body. Humans tend to focus on breathing in, to the extent that they may completely neglect what happens when they breathe out, as if it were not that important. This discrepancy between breathing in and breathing out needs to be corrected in order to create a free-flowing breath. Concentrating on breathing in may fill up the lungs with air all the time, such that the breathing becomes quicker and shorter, and thus stressing both the body and the mind. This may, ironically enough, lead to "feeling out of breath." The wisdom of correct breathing is to empty the lungs of air *completely* so that it may be filled *fully* with air.

Diaphragm breathing

Always use your diaphragm (the diaphragm muscle separating your chest from your abdomen) to breathe, and not your lungs. Essentially, when your diaphragm goes down, you lungs fill up with air; when your diaphragm goes up, your lungs push the air out, expelling the toxic carbon dioxide. Incomplete breathing (when you use your lungs, instead of the diaphragm, to breathe in and breathe out) leads to accumulation of toxic wastes in the lungs and in other parts of your body organs and tissues. Diaphragm breathing is correct breathing to boost health and wellness of both the body and the mind.

Diaphragm breathing is the complete breath. Consciously change your breathing pattern. Use your diaphragm to breathe. Place one hand on your breastbone, feeling that it is raised, and put the other hand above your waist, feeling your diaphragm muscles moving up and down. Deep breathing with your diaphragm gives you complete breath. This is *how* you do your diaphragm breathing:

- Sit comfortably.
- Begin your slow exhalation through your nose.
- Contract your abdomen to empty your lungs.
- Begin your slow inhalation and simultaneously make your belly bulge out.

- Continuing your slow inhalation, now, slightly contract your abdomen and simultaneously lift your chest and hold.
- Continue your slow inhalation, and slowly raise your shoulders. This allows the air to enter fully into your lungs to attain the complete breath.
- Retain your breath and slightly raise your shoulders for a count of 5.
- Very slowly exhale the air. Your upper chest deflates first, and then your abdomen relaxes in.
- Repeat the process.

Learn to slowly prolong your breath, especially your exhalation. Relax your chest and diaphragm muscles, so that you can extend your exhalation, making your breathing out slightly longer and complete. To prolong your exhalation, count "one-and-two-and-three" as you breathe in and breathe out. Make sure that they become balanced. Once you have mastered that, then try to make your breathing out a little longer than your breathing in.

Enhancing Consciousness of Breath

Alternate-nostril breathing

Alternate-nostril breathing is a basic Yoga breathing exercise to balance the right side and the left side of your brain. The left side of your brain governs the right side of your body, including your speech and logical thinking, while the right side of your brain governs the left side of your body, including your creativity and intuition. Achieving balance and harmony between the two sides of your brain is critical and crucial to mind healing for deep relaxation. You can balance your mental energy from the right and the left side of the brain just through practicing this alternate-nostril breathing exercise any time during meditation or any mind-relaxation session. This is *how* you practice alternate-nostril breathing:

- Place your thumb and ring finger lightly on your right and your left nostrils, respectively, with your index and middle fingers resting lightly on your forehead between your eyebrows.
- Exhale deeply through BOTH nostrils.
- Press your thumb against the RIGHT nostril to CLOSE it.
- Breathe in through your LEFT nostril. Count 8.
- CLOSE your LEFT nostril by pressing down your ring finger. Now, BOTH nostrils are closed. Retain the air, and count 4.
- OPEN your RIGHT nostril, and breathe out. Count 8.
- With the LEFT nostril still CLOSED, breathe in through the RIGHT nostril. Count 8.
- CLOSE the RIGHT nostril. Now, BOTH nostrils are closed. Retain the air, and count 4.
- OPEN the LEFT nostril, and breathe out with the RIGHT nostril still closed. Count 8.
- With the RIGHT nostril closed, you have breathed out through the LEFT nostril; you have now completed one round of the breathing exercise.
- Begin the second round by breathing in through the LEFT nostril, and repeat the above.

Here is a summary of alternate-nostril breathing:

- Breathe out through BOTH nostrils. .
- Breathe in through the LEFT nostril (count 8).
- Close BOTH nostrils, and retain air (count 4).

- Breathe out through the RIGHT nostril (count 8).
- Breathe in through the RIGHT nostril (count 8).
- Close BOTH nostrils, and retain air (count 4).
- Breathe out through the LEFT nostril (count 8).
- Breathe in through the LEFT and repeat the whole process.

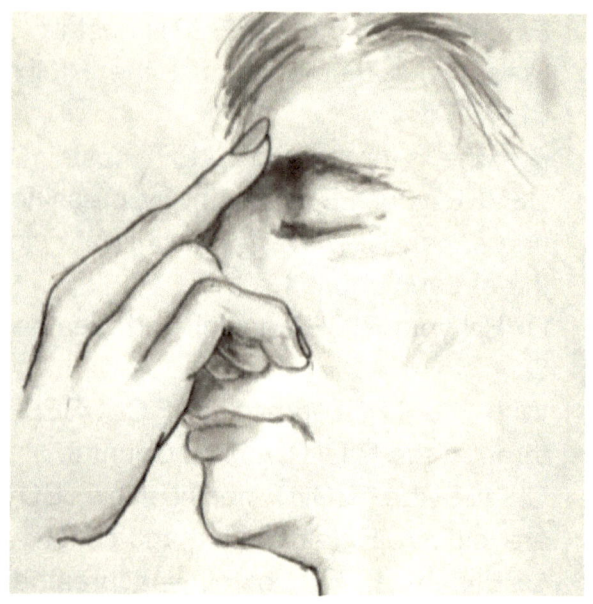

In addition to enhancing your consciousness of breath, alternate-nostril breathing exercise has many other health benefits, including clarity of thinking, deep mental relaxation, awareness and concentration, internal body balance to prevent falls.

Benefits of Consciousness of Breath

Mindfulness

Consciousness of breath is the beginning of mindfulness, which is fixation of the mind on the present moment. When you are conscious of your breath, you subconsciously begin to *slow down* and *notice* how your body reacts to your breathing. Now, you also begin to be aware that your body is yours only and is with you forever, as well as that the present moment is always here and is timeless for you.

This awakening awareness lets you see how your body, mind, and soul are all intricately interconnected with one another to make you feel wholesome. Feeling wholesome enables you become more conscious of what is happening even deep inside your whole being, such as your relationship with others, as well as with the world around you. Once you see your *connectedness* to others and the world, you mind will intuitively know what your body needs, your body will respond to your mind accordingly, and your soul will then oversee the mind with directions and instructions. With this miracle of living, you may become more caring and more compassionate towards others; and you may also have greater clarity of mind to see what is *really* important to you in your life. The result is that you may begin to let go of everything peacefully and willingly—both the desirable and the undesirable, as well as the pleasant and the unpleasant. Mindfulness is profound wisdom that is necessary in the art of living well. Remember, life happens only in the present moment. However, many of us choose to dwell on the past and focus on the future, forgetting that the past was gone and the future is unknown and unpredictable. As a result, we are often distracted by our past thoughts and our future expectations that we become oblivious of what is happening right now, which is the only reality. Mindfulness is makes you feel richer, more down-to-earth, and much more alive, irrespective of your current age and conditions.

With mindfulness of your breath, you will then learn *how* to breathe right, which is complete, natural, and slow. Correct breathing means you get more oxygen to your lungs, cells, and organs, and thus leading to better health.

If you are mindful of your breath, you will also become mindful of your eating, you will not simply shuffle and stuff food into your mouth without savoring each morsel of food in your mouth.

Posture

Consciousness of breath is optimal breathing, which ultimately affects your body posture. Good posture means in any standing position, you body posture should be as follows:

- Your head is directly above your shoulders. Your ear, shoulder, and hip are in a straight line from a side view.
- Your upper back is straight, not slouched.
- Your shoulders blades, relaxed and straight, are flat against your back.
- Your pelvis is in a neutral position (lined up vertically, not slanted)
- Your knees are unlocked.

Consciousness holds the key to maintaining your good standing posture, which affects your breathing.

<u>Steps for good standing posture</u>

- Stand with your feet hip-width apart (for better balance).

- Align your ears, shoulders, and hips (Using a mirror for alignment, if necessary).
- Unlock both of your knees (maintaining "neutral" pelvis; avoiding your pelvis from tilting forward).
- Pull in your abdominal muscles.
- Inhale naturally.
- Exhale slowly while pulling your belly button into the spine.
- Lift your rib cage (straightening your rounded upper back; while expanding your lungs for deeper breathing).
- Realign your head over your shoulders (your head not leaning backwards).
- Pull in your abdominal muscles.
- Inhale naturally.
- Un-round your shoulders (by rotating your arms until your palms facing your thighs).
- Gently press your shoulders down, away from your ears.
- Pull your shoulder blades towards the spine.
- Stretch your head upwards without tilting backwards.

It is highly recommended for men to wear suspenders, instead of belts. The explanation is that, whether you have belly fat or not, if you tuck in your tummy, you may have a tendency to "drop" your pants, so you tend to push your tummy "forward" instead of tucking it in—this is how you might have your bad body posture in the first place.

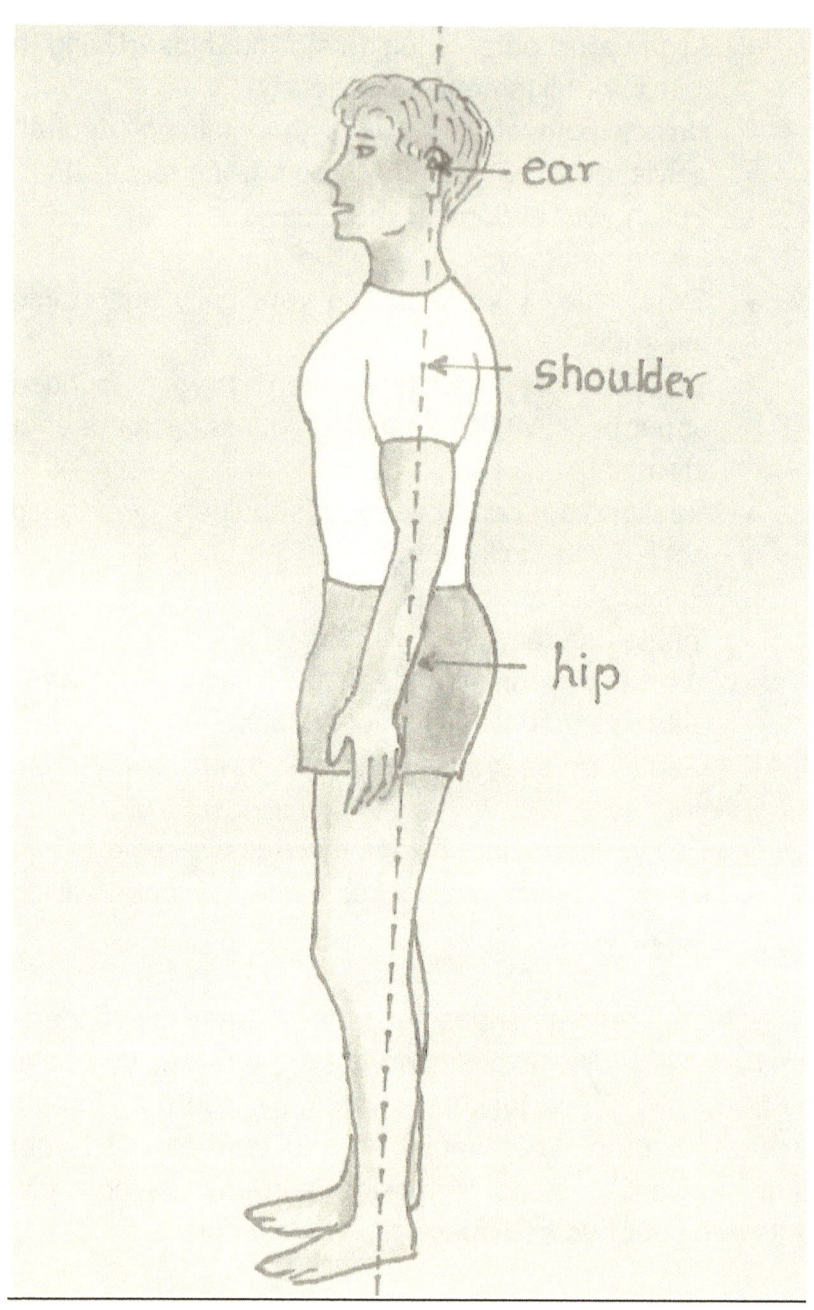

Exercise for good standing posture

- Stand with your back against a wall with heels several inches away from the wall.
- Relax your arms.
- Slowly bend your knees, while pressing the small of your back against the wall.
- Lift your rib cage and press the back of your head to the wall.
- Press the back of your shoulders to the wall, while you pull your shoulder blades together.
- Hold the position.
- Press your back and shoulders to the wall.
- Bend your knees and slide down the wall.
- Slide back up the wall.
- Relax and repeat.

Maintain your good standing posture through constant consciousness. With more practice, you will still be able to change your posture even in your advanced years.

Remember, good standing posture not only enhances your breathing but also makes you look and feel younger. You have seen many seniors walking with a crooked back, much like the hunchback of Notre Dame. A slumped upper back has many drawbacks: it decreases the capacity of your lungs, resulting in shallow breathing; it presses your rib cage downwards, thereby exerting pressure on your heart, liver, and stomach; and it makes you look much older and shorter. But you don't have to be like that if you are conscious of your standing and walking posture at all times.

Detoxification

According to **Dr. Andrew Weil**, the benefits of deep

conscious breathing cannot be under-emphasized. By focusing on the breath, and by practicing deep breathing, we may give the body an internal cleansing by pumping more oxygen into the lungs and bloodstream, thereby instrumental in creating more white blood cells, as well as empowering the lymphatic system for detoxification. Dr. Andrew Weil recommends the following:

- Place the tip of your tongue against the ridge behind your upper teeth and exhale completely through your mouth so that you make a "whoosh" sound.
- Close your mouth and inhale deeply through your nose for a count 4, hold your breath for 7 counts, and then exhale through your mouth for a count of 8.
- Repeat at least three or four times.

If You Just Don't Die

The bottom line: correct breathing is a blessing in life. It gives one a sense of delight, stimulation, and even inspiration. As a matter of fact, the word "inspiration" comes from the Latin word *inspirare*, which means "breathing in." When you inhale, you receive, and when you exhale, you give away. You cannot receive without giving out, and one is impossible without the other. They are opposites that are forever linked together, just like the *yin* and the *yang* in classical Chinese cosmology. This is a strong testament to the wisdom of letting go: giving up to receive more. It is always more blessed to give than to receive, just as it is more beneficial to have an exhalation longer than an inhalation.

THREE

CONSCIOUSNESS OF THINKING

"The conscious mind may be compared to a fountain playing in the sun and falling back into the great subterranean pool of subconscious from which it rises." **Sigmund Freud**

If you have become conscious of your breath, most probably you have also become conscious of many other things in life, including consciousness of your thoughts. Living is consciousness in that you must always be aware that your mind does not get in your own way, especially if you just don't die and have to continue the rest of your life journey.

Consciousness of the Subconscious

The human mind is intelligent in that it inherently knows how to organize life experiences into different patterns so that they may be easily and readily available. These thinking patterns are just like a filing cabinet with its many different drawers and many different folders, each with a different tag to indicate what that is. That filing cabinet has become the subconscious of the individual who has created it; whenever looking for information, that individual would automatically go and search through the many drawers and folders in his or her filing cabinet.

Implicit assumptions

We all have our own individual *automatic* thinking patterns to help us organize our thoughts, just like looking through our own filing cabinet, and thus enabling us to make our subjective observations, generalizations, predictions, and expectations. Automatically, they may have become the many implicit assumptions to help us see how life works or doesn't work for us.

Indeed, we are living in an assumptive world with just too many implicit assumptions that may often become stumbling blocks in our lives—in particular, in *how* we think. Consciousness of the subconscious may help us see the ultimate truth in our own implicit assumptions—the truth that nothing is set in stone, and that we can still teach an old dog new tricks. The truth of the matter is that we have to *rethink* our minds in order to believe that there are many exceptions to all our assumptions derived from our own observations, leading to our many generalizations and expectations that we may have subconsciously created for ourselves. Our consciousness of the subconscious may help us live the rest of our lives very *differently*, and not as what we may have erroneously assumed.

Always use your consciousness to look deeply into what is *really* happening in your thinking mind—or *how* it might have got in your own way by providing you with superficial observations leading to over-generalizations that are often followed by automatic predictions and expectations in your implicit assumptive world. Let your consciousness deliver you from the half-truths and untruths you might have been floundering in all these years.

As an illustration, your daughter is about to get married; she plans to have a family soon; she is looking for a house to buy—*that* she will be happily married is based on your automatic thinking pattern of implicit assumptions. But the reality is that there might be many exceptions to all your assumptions: the marriage might be canceled at the last moment; the pregnancy might be unsuccessful; the new home might be destroyed in a wildfire, a hurricane, or a tornado, and so on and so forth.

Life is full of changes, and many of which are sudden and unpredictable—they often become the exceptions to your implicit assumptions. With consciousness of thinking, you may find more exceptions to all your automatic assumptions; with more exceptions, you may then become not only less resistant but also more adaptable to any unpredictable change that you may encounter or experience along your life journey. Don't let your automatic assumptions limit what you will be able to see and experience in life. If you just don't die, the sky is the limit.

Always challenge and change your assumptions; they are no more than your selective attention to what you want to believe. Over the years, have you been looking for jobs that do not challenge your expectations? Do you always select your favorite news channel based on your assumptive expectations?

Maybe, now is the time to do what you normally don't do—or what is known as *reverse thinking*.

Reverse thinking

Reverse thinking is what the ancient Chinese sage, **Lao Tzu** (老子), suggested in his immortal classic, *Tao Te Ching* (道德經), a book of poetry on human wisdom.

According to Lao Tzu, reverse thinking begins with an empty mindset, which lets go of any implicit assumption so that there may be room for clarity of thinking to understand how your implicit assumptions can create predictions and expectations in your assumptive world that never become your realities. Reverse thinking is the antidote to any pre-conditioned thinking, which is implicit assumption based on subjective predictions and expectations.

Consciousness may free yourself from the shackles of any automatic assumptive thinking that might have enslaved you, keeping you in bondage without your knowing it. Are you the master, or just a slave of your own life? Often times, we think we are masters of our lives and we are in total control, but in fact we are no more than slaves. You are the master only when you have complete control over your life, or rather over your way of thinking. Remember, your subconscious mind controls you with all your implicit assumptions. They make you act, react in different situations and circumstances in life. With reverse thinking, you may see more exceptions to whatever your pre-conditioned mind sees and says.

Consciousness of the Happiness Mindset

Happiness is the essence of life and living. Therefore, almost each and every one of us is always in quest of happiness because it is the meaning of our existence. In addition, advertising, consumerism, and the media have all mesmerized us into believing that happiness is one of the basic human rights we are all entitled to.

The reality is that Americans are becoming poorer, and many are living from hand to mouth. Scientists have been asking for decades the exact same question about the degree of personal happiness to an individual, and those who say they are happy are getting fewer.

The different perceptions of happiness

Happiness is all in the mind. You have to be conscious of *why* you are happy or unhappy.

You have both a conscious and a subconscious mind. Simply put, your conscious mind does all your active thinking: selectively recording whatever data and information you want to remember, while purposely discarding whatever you consciously think is irrelevant or inapplicable to you. Your subconscious mind, on the other hand, absorbs everything indiscriminately that you are exposed to, and stores it at the back of your subconscious mind in the form of assumptions, emotions, feelings, and memories—they all have become the raw materials with which you weave the fabrics of the realities of your life, making you happy or unhappy, depending on how you perceive and relate them to your personality and life experiences. That is why you have to be conscious of your thinking in order to change your mind in order to change your perceptions of personal happiness—whether it is a glass half-full or a glass half-empty.

The different happiness mindsets

In general, there are four different happiness mindsets. Not only the characteristics of one type of mindset may overlap those of another, but also one type of mindset may become another; it is all in the consciousness of thinking.

The unhappy ones

There are those who are forever unhappy due to an unhappy childhood, an unfulfilled adult life, and many unhappy life experiences throughout the life journey. They have made indelible imprints on their minds, making them see only problems, instead of potentials ahead of them. They don't want to live, but they just don't die. Not wanting or knowing how to purposely end their lives, they just drift on, or simply live a reckless life in hope of an early demise.

They have suffered and gone through too much in their lives. They don't know how to cope with their life problems and how to deal with their life challenges. They have despaired and become helpless. They are forever the unhappy ones because unhappiness has become their brain chemicals.

The neither-happy-nor-unhappy ones

There are those who have always been a spectator, instead of a participant, of life; they are forever sitting on the sidelines of life, observing others and never thinking they could be a part of it. They always believe that life is not worth taking chances because their minds have been filled with many assumptions that they are not competent enough to get involved. Inactivity and passivity play a major role in their lives. They may not like their current situations, but they don't know how and where to start to change them. Even if they have the know-how, they don't want to do it, or unless someone would do it for them. Life is too much for them; they just stay back and stay put, not taking any chance or exerting any effort, while they try to get by with whatever they have. They never see the need to take the initiative to create a better life for themselves.

If they just don't die, they just carry on with their lives with episodes of high and low, always wondering why they don't have what they wish they had, or why others are always having what they don't have.

The to-be-happy ones

There are those who are always in quest of happiness. But, unfortunately, they are like a mule in front of a carrot-and-stick: the more pain inflicted on the mule, the more desirous the mule wants to reach out for the forever unreachable carrot in front. Their desirable but unattainable happiness is forever in front of them.

They have the problematic mindset of "better" and "more" in their endless quest for careers, relationships, and material comforts that have become the objectives of their personal happiness. Their to-be-happiness just keeps them always wanting "better" and "more" in order to feel happy.

The happy ones

There are those who have the wisdom to understand that true happiness requires action and effort, that happiness is only a moment-to-moment feeling, and that happiness never lasts.

Happiness is *feeling good* about yourself, and it requires you to take some action in order to feel good about yourself. Remember, elated feelings, such as happiness, satisfaction, and fulfillment, are not the natural and normal resting states of the human mind, therefore, you must take a *deliberate* action in order to achieve and activate those innate mental states.

Our ancestors in the Stone Age did not naturally and instinctively feel comfortable, secure, and satisfied with their status quo. They certainly did not pass those genes on to us. They had to fight to survive; by the same token, we all must make a conscious effort to take some action in order to feel good, happy, and satisfied.

Remember, true human happiness is a process, a way of living, involving some action to change the consciousness of thinking. It is no more than the ability to experience joy when good things happen; the ability to feel satisfaction when goals are achieved; the ability to cope with problems, the ability to adapt to changes, and the ability to give meaning and purpose to life.

Consciousness of the Choice of Thoughts

According to **Descartes**, the great French philosopher, your mind thinks, and you create your thoughts, which are then expressed in language or words. You can choose your words, just as you can choose your thoughts.

As a simple illustration, here are some plain facts about my grandfather:

> He came from China to the United States at the end of the 19th century. He studied at Cornell University, where he earned his bachelor's degree in economics. He became a successful banker, and started his own banking business in New York City. He made a great fortune, and began investing in real estate, making millions of dollars Then came the Great Depression, and he lost everything because he had to pay tax for all his real estate investments.

With an implicit presumptive mindset, my predictive

thoughts with expectations could be: "If it hadn't been for the Great Depression, he might have become a real estate billionaire. He could have left my father—his only son—a great fortune, and we would have been very rich. . . . . .How unfair that he had to pay all the land and real estate taxes that bankrupted him!"

With a different mindset, my thoughts could be: "Wealth and good fortune are unpredictable, and nothing in this material world is permanent. So, we should be grateful for whatever we presently have."

We all have a *choice* when we process data and information in our minds: with consciousness, we can always add or delete our own assumptions, expectations, and predictions. Again, with consciousness, we can choose to think about it, or simply reject it. For example, if my thoughts about my grandfather tend to be negative, then I could reject them whenever they pop up in my mind; on the hand, if my thoughts about my grandfather are positive, then I could share the story of my grandfather with my friends.

The bottom line: we all have a *choice* about what is happening in our minds. If an unpleasant past experience pops up in the brain, make a conscious effort to distract it by thinking about something else instead. We all have a choice.

If You Just Don't Die

If you just don't die and continue to live to a ripe old age, you will certainly have many unpleasant experiences that might have left many indelible imprints in your mind. These negative memories will continue to show up every now and then, especially when you are all alone by yourself. Therefore, it is important to be always conscious of their presence, as well as conscious of how these thoughts may affect your thinking. Remember, they belonged to the past, which was gone forever. Even positive memories with positive emotions might turn negative, if you compare them with your present situation.

The bottom line: let go of all thoughts related to the past; instead, always be conscious of the present. .

FOUR

CONSCIOUSNESS OF WELLNESS

"Wellness is the complete integration of body, mind, and spirit—the realization that everything we do, think, feel, and believe has an effect on our state of well-being." **Greg Anderson**

Consciousness of Body-Mind Connection

Your body lives in the physical world, and thus it plays a pivotal role in your overall being, including your mind and your soul. Science has already attested to the close connection between the body and the mind: the body affects the mind as much as the mind affects the body.

Human emotions, in particular, affect the physical body. In **Woody Allen**'s movie *Annie Hall*, **Diane Keaton** would like to know why he wasn't angry. "I don't get angry," he humorously replied, "I grow a tumor instead." Indeed, toxic emotions can lead to a toxic body.

According to Traditional Chinese Medicine (TCM),

human emotions are the major underlying causes of many diseases and disorders because for centuries Chinese physicians have believed that certain body organs are related to emotional activities; for example, the heart is related to joy, the liver to anger, the spleen to obsessive thoughts, the lungs to anxiety, and the kidneys to fear. Therefore, excessive emotions may disrupt the free flow of *qi*, the life-giving energy that flows through the body, and thus causing imbalance and disharmony that may lead to diseases and disorders.

In addition, human behaviors—often a byproduct of human emotions—affect the mind, just as emotions of the mind affecting the body. According to a study at Ohio State University in 2003, physical behavior, such as enhanced body language of nodding in agreement or shaking head in disagreement, may significantly affect how we think without our knowing it. According to that study, even posture, such as sitting up straight, may be conducive to remembering positive memories or thinking positively, because posture changes the production of human hormones.

The interconnection between the body and the mind is further evidenced by the indisputable notion that a healthy heart produces a healthy brain by pumping sufficient oxygen and nutrients to nourish the brain through its bloodstream.

Consciousness of Physical Wellness

At the physical level, your wellness is basically affected by what you eat, what you drink, and what you do with your body. It's just that simple; its complexity is no more than distractions from your consciousness of doing the right things for your physical body.

Just be conscious of the right numbers: your body weight, your blood pressure, and your cholesterol levels. If you take good care of these numbers, which are inter-related, the rest of will take care of themselves. There is only one indisputable fact, with no exception: a centenarian is never obese. If you wish to live longer, not necessarily to one hundred years and beyond, you must do something about your body weight *now*, and not later.

Body weight

Your body weight determines your body shape, which defines your body image, which is a reflection of your physical wellness.

An ideal body weight is anti-aging. In fact, your body shape is already a reflection of your overall health. Good weight management is critical to remaining younger and healthier for longer. As a matter of fact, it is so important that Americans are spending billions of dollars every year just to keep them in better shape. Sadly, many are lost in this battle of the bulge.

To lose weight, you need determination, discipline, and perseverance. There are no short cuts, no cutting corners, and no magic bullets, such as weight-loss diets that aim at ripping off your cash and not your fat or extra pounds.

Eating *less* holds the key to weight loss. Weight loss is all about calories, and not about *counting* calories. Eat only when you are hungry. Do not eat for the sake of eating (that is, when it is meal time), to satisfy your emotional needs (eating disorders), or to gratify your urge (food cravings) for certain foods. To lose weight permanently, you simply *eat less*.

Eat *naturally*. To eat naturally, do not go on any fad diet, such as the Atkins Diet or the South Beach Diet. Remember, any diet is *abnormal* eating, which will upset your natural relationship with foods, leading to food cravings, or an eating disorder, such as anorexia or binge eating, further down the road. In addition, any diet will affect your body's metabolism. If, for any reason, you have to give up that diet, you may have a dysfunctional metabolism, leading to immediate weight gain or weight fluctuation. To eat naturally, avoid all processed foods, which are loaded with chemicals, such as food colorings, food enhancers, and preservatives. All processed foods are designed to make you "feel" hungry and want to eat more. The consumer is always the ultimate loser—losing both health and money, except those extra pounds!

Body mass

Studies have shown that weight training in doing leg presses and squats not just improves your leg muscles—it boosts your body's natural production of youth hormones to increase not only your muscle mass and strength but also your mental alertness.

Astronauts in weightlessness in space tend to lose more calcium in their bones due to the absence of gravitational weight on their bones. Therefore, weight training enhances bone density, making your bones younger for longer.

Weight training can be performed with state-of-the-art equipment, or just simply using dumbbells to do your daily routines and exercises to get the same results. The choice is yours.

The importance of muscles

Your muscles not only keep you in shape but also maintain your health and wellness. They are essential for life. Muscle protein is dynamic when it is converted into amino acids. It repairs your body cells and tissues. It helps you fight infections. It carries oxygen (in the form of hemoglobin) to your cells. It transports calcium and iron in your blood. It controls your weight (your muscles burn calories even while you sleep—one pound of muscle burns 30 to 40 calories a day).

Having more muscles means getting less fat. Muscles reduce inflammation (excess fat producing more cytokines, responsible for artery, joint, and tissue inflammation). Inflammation leads to plague formation in arteries (risk of heart disease). Muscles provide body strength and mobility, and thus reducing the risk of developing diabetes later in life.

Your muscles are important. Use them or lose them!

A study on master athletes at the University of California indicated that muscle mass has little to do with age. In other words, you could still have the same amount of muscle mass as someone who is 10 to 20 years younger than you are. Muscle mass is anti-aging. Do weight training or workout without weights to preserve your muscle mass and keep you in shape to look forever younger.

Women, in particular, benefit more from weight training, because they have less muscle mass than men have, and adding more muscles means burning more calories.

Loss of muscle mass

As you age, you muscle protein dwindles. An average person loses half a pound of muscles and gains a pound of fat a year. Between 30 and 60, you may expect to lose 15 pounds of muscles and gain 30 pounds of fat (if not more). That will put you not only out of shape, but also in health hazards.

Loss of muscle mass may be due to the following:

- Increase in cortisol (a hormone for regulating your blood sugar, blood pressure, immune function, and inflammatory response), which breaks down muscle mass
- Decrease in growth hormone (stimulating growth and cell reproduction) and testosterone (male and female hormone)
- Increase in fat (more fat, more inflammation, and less muscle mass—a vicious cycle)

To prevent loss of muscle mass, continue to build your muscles even as you age. The human body is perfectly capable of getting the exercise it needs with no extra equipment. For instance, even a simple towel can be used as one of the most effective and versatile fitness accessories for strength and flexibility training to enhance your muscle mass.

Important muscle groups

As you age, weight training should specifically target the following muscle groups for prolonged independence and continuous mobility:

- Back, knee, pelvic floor (important for your sexual function, bowel and urinary control)
- Shoulder joint and shoulder rotator cuff to stabilize shoulder movements

Remember, exercise, not medications, is the single most effective choice against heart disease. Always exercise your muscles.

Balance and harmony

For thousands of years, the Chinese have observed the importance of balance and harmony, manifested in the concept of the "yin" and the "yang" (represented as the *female* and *male*, respectively, or any two opposite yet complementary energy states in the universe). A balance between the two polarities can help you stay in beneficial energy alignment, which is fundamental to your wellness and well-being. The "yin" embodies negative electrical charge and contractive energy, while the "yang" demonstrates positive electrical charge and expansive energy. Your health is contingent on the balance of the "yin" and the "yang" within you.

The balance of the "yin" and the "yang" is reflected in the Five Elements.

The Five Elements

The Chinese concept of balance and harmony originates from the Five Elements (wood, fire, earth, metal, and water), which not only are fundamental to the cycles of Nature, but also correspond to the different organs of the human body. In addition, each of these Five Elements also corresponds to a different color in food.

The Five Elements not only balance but also complement each other to create internal harmony, which holds the key to physical wellness. To illustrate, water nourishes trees or wood; without wood, there will be no fire (which burns wood); without fire burning wood, there will be no earth (the ashes from the burnt wood); without earth, there will be no metal (from the earth itself); through condensation, fire heats metal to produce water; without metal, there will be no water; without water, there will be no tree or wood. These Five Elements are therefore interdependent on one another for their existence in the form of a cycle of Nature.

Wood corresponding to green

Eat green vegetables, from asparagus to dark leafy greens, such as spinach. Eat green fruits, such as lime and melon. Eat pumpkin seeds. Eat green-colored beans, such as lentils, and mung beans; and green grains, such as rye.

Fire corresponding to red

Eat red vegetables, such as hot red peppers and bell peppers, or beets. Eat red fruits, such as red apples, or cherries. Eat red nuts, such as pecans. Eat red-colored beans, such as red lentils, red beans; and red grains, such as buckwheat.

Earth corresponding to orange and yellow

Eat orange and yellow vegetables, such as pumpkins, squash, and yams. Eat orange and yellow fruits, such as mangoes, oranges, and papaya. Eat orange and yellow nuts, such as almonds and cashews. Eat orange and yellow beans, such as chickpeas, orange and yellow grains, such as corn, and millet.

Metal corresponding to white

Eat white vegetables, such as cauliflower, and daikon radish. Eat white fruits, such as bananas, and pears. Eat white nuts, such as macadamias, and pine nuts. Eat white-colored beans, such as soybeans, white beans; and white grains, such as rice, and barley.

Water corresponding to black, blue, and purple

Eat dark-colored vegetables, such as black mushroom, eggplant, and seaweed. Eat dark-colored fruits, such as blackberries, blueberries, and raisins. Eat dark-colored nuts, such as black sesame, and walnuts. Eat dark-colored beans, such as black beans, navy beans; and dark-colored grains, such as black wild rice.

According to the famous *Yellow Emperor's Classic of Medicine*, health and longevity are contingent on a balance and harmony of all the five elemental energies. Therefore, you are recommended to eat a diet that includes vegetables, fruits, nuts, beans, and grains of all the five colors to make sure you would live to a ripe old age, if you just don't die.

Body chemistry

Your aging body cells need an optimum environment for replication and rejuvenation. They need a balanced acid-and-alkaline environment (known as pH).

Acid and alkaline are substances that have opposing qualities. Your body functions at its best when the pH is optimum, which is slightly alkaline. The pH of your blood, tissues, and body fluids directly affects the state of your overall cellular health. Your diet is the primary source that determines the acid-alkaline levels in your body.

The pH level

The pH scale ranges between one and fourteen. *Seven* is considered neutral. Anything *below* seven is considered *acidic*, while anything *above* seven is considered *alkaline*. Deviations above or below a 7.30 and 7.40 pH range can signal potentially serious and even dangerous symptoms, forewarning you of a disease in process. Measure the acid and alkaline levels in your body by performing a simple urine test with litmus paper obtainable from your local pharmacy.

Over-acidification

Acidification often comes from excess intake of foods containing great amounts of acid; insufficient elimination by the body through the kidneys (urination) and the skin (sweating). Not too much acid can actually stay in the bloodstream, and, accordingly, any excess is directed to other body organs and tissues, where it can accumulate.

Over-acidification can make your body sick. When your body is too acidic, your cell tissues are forced to relinquish their alkaline reserves, depleting them of alkaline minerals, which are some of the essential components of the tissues themselves. In addition, the corrosive nature of acid irritates your body organs, causing inflammation (which is often a source of body pain among the elderly), aches, and hardening of tissues. Acidic sweat may cause skin allergy, especially in areas where sweat seems to accumulate, such as the armpits. Acidic urine may also cause infection and inflammation in the urinary tract, resulting in many bladder problems. Over-acidification not only causes lesions of the mucous membrane in your respiratory system, making them more vulnerable to infections, but also impairs your immune system.

Acid foods contain a good deal of acid, and are acidic in taste, and they include some of the following: blueberries, blackberries, raspberries, and strawberries; grapefruits and oranges, lemons and tangerines; sweet fruits, such as watermelon; unripe fruits; acid vegetable, such as rhubarb, tomato, and watercress; honey; vinegar; and yogurt. (Please note that many fruits contain acids but have an alkaline effect on the body.)

Always eat the fruit, instead of drinking its juice. The reason is that alkaline minerals are present in the pulp; the juice without the pulp is only more acidic. Cooking the fruit does not remove its acidity.

Acid foods, however, may be alkalizing if the metabolism of your body is efficient. In other words, if your body can easily metabolize and oxidize them, these foods can be transformed into alkaline elements, making your body more alkaline, instead of more acidic.

Alkalizing the body

You can reduce or eliminate over-acidification in your body by changing your lifestyle, making it less stressful, by adjusting your diet for more alkaline foods and drinks, by consuming medicinal plants, such as black currant and cranberry, to promote the flow of urine (diuretics) and to improve the production of sweat by exercise, and by taking alkaline mineral supplements to facilitate your internal cleansing.

Alkalizing foods contain little or no acid substances, and they do not produce acids when metabolized by your body. Alkalizing foods include all green vegetables, colored vegetables (except tomato), chestnuts, potatoes, avocados, bananas, black olives, dried fruits, almonds and Brazil nuts, cold-pressed oils, and alkaline mineral water.

As you age, health is everything—just as **Dr. Deepak Chopra**, M.D., bestselling author, founder of the Chopra Center for Wellbeing, says: "If you don't take care of your health today, you will be forced to take care of your illness tomorrow."

A balanced acid-alkaline level increases your energy and

vitality, neutralizes excess acids in your body, removes accumulated toxins in your blood, strengthens your weakened immune system and organ systems, destroys harmful microorganisms, and balances your overall body chemistry.

If you have insomnia, mood swings, chronic fatigue, aches and pain, dull skin, brittle hair and nails, difficulty in concentration, and other health issues, you do not have a balanced acid-alkaline level in your body.

Optimize your body's acid-and-alkaline level with your diet. Here is a list of common foods in regard to their acid and alkaline levels for general reference:

Acid foods

Rice bran, dried fish, egg yolk, oatmeal, brown rice, tuna, chicken, pearl barley, oysters, salmon, buckwheat, scallops, pork, peanuts, beef, cheese, whole barley, shrimp, peas, beer, bread, butter, asparagus

Alkaline foods

Seaweed, ginger, kidney beans, shitake mushrooms, mushrooms, spinach, soybeans, bananas, chestnuts, carrots, strawberries, potatoes, cabbage, radish, squash, sweet potatoes, turnips, orange juice, apples, egg white, coffee, tea, cucumber, onions, string beans

Remember, some of the acid-forming foods may become alkaline if the acids are properly metabolized by the body. The goal is to attain balance.

Consciousness of Mental Wellness

Mental wellness is as important as, if not more important

than, physical wellness.

Do you have mental wellness?

The essentials of mental wellness

You may not have mental wellness if you have depression, or you are regularly suffering from episodes of unexplained sadness.

You may not have mental wellness if your love relationships are always under stress and strain, and your children are forever rebellious and uncontrollable.

You may not have mental wellness if you are always on the verge of good health and success, but you never quite seem to be getting them.

You may not have mental wellness if you have achieved some accomplishments in your life, and yet you are forever plagued by frustration, and never quite seem to be enjoying the fruits of your success.

You may not have mental wellness if you find yourself struggling with something that you can neither identify nor understand.

You may not have mental wellness if you always feel a long, evil arm stretching from the past, trying to grip hold of you, and pulling you back from reaching your life goals and realizing your dreams.

All of us may have some problems with our mental wellness to a greater or lesser extent because we are all living in a toxic world that may somehow and somewhat affect our mental health and wellness. You are not the exception. Our minds may have become saturated with toxic thoughts and memories. You *know* you have a toxic mind when you are always wrestling with a dark shadow or a darker side of you that you cannot quite explain or get rid of.

Therefore, it is important to be conscious of your mental

wellness so as to improve it, instead of letting it deteriorate further.

Mental wellness begins with the thinking mind. Never think with your assumptions without their exceptions; never think with your hopes, wishes, or fears without validating their authenticity. Always think with clarity of mind, which is thinking without your emotions.

According to Traditional Chinese Medicine (TCM), there are seven emotions that disharmonize the body and the mind: anger, fear, fright, grief, joy, worry, and pensiveness or over-concentration. At first glance, "joy" may seem to be the only positive emotion among the seven negative ones. However, at close scrutiny, even "joy" may also become toxic, especially in an inflated ego. A case in point, the once-celebrated-but-now-disgraced cyclist **Lance Armstrong** used performance-enhancing drugs to win his races in order to sustain and protect his ego of winning to give him "joy" that led to his ultimate downfall in his career.

Toxic emotions may also easily lead to the Seven Deadly Sins of lust, gluttony, greed, sloth, wrath, envy, and pride. Toxic thoughts originating from toxic emotions may become toxic memories stored in the back of the subconscious mind. Toxic memories may then cause the conscious mind to make toxic choices and decisions, leading to toxic behaviors, actions and reactions, that further exacerbate the mental wellness of an individual.

Thoughts and memories may make you "think" you are who you have now become; they are the raw materials with which you have created your ego-self. But what you "think" you have now become may not be the "real" you. That is why you need to "rethink" your mind in order to find out who you really are, and not who you think or wish you were.

Rethink the mind

To enhance your mental wellness, you need to *rethink* your mind. Your thoughts may not be what they seem to be; do not let them deceive or mislead you. Even your so-called "reality" is only created by your memories as well as by your projections of those memories into the future, deluding yourself into thinking that they are for real. Nothing could be further from the truth. Therefore, you must, so to speak, *listen* with mindfulness to your thoughts; *understand* with consciousness how they may affect your feelings and emotions, as well as your actions and reactions; and then *validate* them with non-judgmental objectivity. They are some of the essentials of rethinking your mind. **Albert Einstein** once said: "The world we have created is a product of our thinking; it cannot be changed without changing our thinking." Therefore, to change the reality, you must change your mind *first*—or rather, stop your thinking mind from being controlled by your assumptions and presumptions.

Thoughts, which ultimately become memories, can be as dangerous and devastating as assault weapons, if they are mishandled. Banish your toxic thoughts from your mind *before* they become your toxic memories and realities, generating negative chemicals in your brain.

Understand that a thought generated by a past memory is *real* to you. It is not imaginary, but as real as life to *you* alone. Your thought sends a message to your brain, which then begins to process the signal, and releases certain brain chemicals. You then become *aware* of your own thinking. No matter what you think, your thought is real to *you*, and must be treated as *real*. The goal is to be *conscious* of the thought and then *change* your perception of that thought accordingly.

Be conscious of your body's reactions to the chemicals released by your brain as a thought occurs. For example, if you are angry, *notice* how your muscles tense up and how your heart beats faster than normal. Train yourself to *notice* the differences in your body's different reactions to different thoughts that come up in your mind.

Do not base on a memory to predict the future, to read into someone's mind, or to explain someone's actions and intentions. In other words, do not anticipate or speculate what is going on in the mind of another person, if you cannot even control what is going on in your own mind.

According to a research team from Lund University in Sweden, actively, deliberately, and repeatedly trying to forget an unwanted memory can help you actually erase that memory from your subconscious mind. That is to say, if you consciously repress a memory long enough, you can forget it completely.

Subliminal messages

Subliminal messages are positive messages sent directly to your subconscious mind, which controls your conscious mind. Use subliminal messages to *consciously control* what you may be doing all day long and everyday—thinking *uncreatively* and *unintelligently*. **Albert Einstein** once said: "Any man who reads too much and uses his own brain too little falls into lazy habits of thinking." Maybe you should start using your brain more often to create more subliminal messages for your mental wellness.

Subliminal messages are powerful mental tools to enhance your mind power. Empower your mind with subliminal messages, which work as a mild form of self-hypnosis—slowly and gradually sending suggestions into your subconscious mind to subtly change any incorrect self-beliefs, wrong ways of thinking, and even undesirable patterns of behavior. These subliminal messages allow you not only to bypass your "logical" conscious mind but also to overcome any resistance that may hold you back, thereby enabling you to access your subconscious mind with positive messages for mind empowerment. Subliminal messages are powerful tools to empower your mind to live a much better and more meaningful life even in your old age.

Once you have mastered the subliminal messages, you can master your mind by controlling its thoughts. Remember, you are your thoughts, and your life is a byproduct of your thoughts. As **Napoleon Hill**, the famous writer, said: "What the mind of man can conceive and believe, it can achieve." Yes, you can achieve success in your second career, weight loss, relationships, or just about anything you have set your mind on. The possibilities are limitless at any age.

How to use subliminal messages

You can use subliminal messages to erase unwanted memories. In order to be effective, subliminal messages have to be in the first person "I", and must be in the present tense. For example, "I am letting go of this memory", "I am overcoming the feeling of anger from this memory" and "I am forgiving myself and others as well." In addition, subliminal messages have to be repeated as often as possible, and with a relaxed mind in order to be beneficial and effective. Create your own subliminal messages and repeat them as often as necessary. Always *talk back* with subliminal messages to any negative thought generated by a past memory, especially a toxic one.

You must use words about yourself and not someone else. Always use "I" in your subliminal messages because they are all about *you* and not someone else, for example, "I am happy!" You must use the present tense as if you are speaking to your mind right now, for example, "I am healthy and strong!"

You must prompt your subconscious mind to remember the things you want, not the things you don't. For example, do not say: "I am now going to give up alcohol!" because your subconscious mind registers "alcohol" which is what you would want to give up; instead, say: "I am now going to be sober!"

You must always be positive, and not the reverse of a negative, such as, "I am *not* old and decrepit."

You must repeat your subliminal messages when you are mentally relaxed, and you must repeat them consistently and diligently to achieve the desired effect.

Visualization

Visualization is another powerful mental tool to help you achieve your goals in controlling your mind. Visualize your future self in your mind's eye. A picture is worth a thousand words. If you can imagine it, you can achieve it.

Harness the power of visualization to make it more "real" to you, and this gives you the incentive to pursue your goals in any stage of your life. Visualization is manifestation of your desires by vibrating their mental energy frequencies in a positive way.

How to visualize

You must be very relaxed; your mind must be in a deep level of relaxation. You must "strongly feel" that you have already got what you want, not just "thinking" about getting what you want. Remember, "wanting" is the opposite of "having." The former generates negative energy frequencies, while the latter creates positive ones. Positive feelings are a key component of visualization.

You must visualize with specific details to authenticate

the reality of your visualization. For example, when visualizing how you are going to drive your golf ball to a distant target, see in your mind's eye how you swing your golf club, how your shoulders rotate, how your torso moves as you bring down the golf club to strike the ball, and how the golf ball flies into the air to that intended distant target. Give as many details to your visualization.

You must be in full control. A positive image stems from an internal focus of control, which means you always act instead of reacting, and you are always the master of a situation, instead of the victim, worrying about its possible negative outcome.

You must be consistent in your visualization. Your mind is a muscle; you must exercise it constantly and consistently to create the desirable strength to accomplish its mission.

You must be patient with your visualization. You must think long term; that is, you must patiently wait for the manifestation of your goals visualized.

Changing attitudes

If you don't like something, then change it. If you can't change it, then change your attitude or perception. An attitude is no more than a thought empowered by words and images. In life, every thought counts because your whole being is composed of thoughts. Research studies have demonstrated the importance of mind power in that thoughts can even turn on or turn off a particular gene responsible for a particular disease or disorder. In other words, your thoughts may impact your health, as well as everything else in your life.

Utilize your mind power to develop the right attitudes for positive and longevity living. The key to dynamic living is having positive thinking, which can bring about physical and mental transformation, as well as emotional and spiritual unfolding in your life journey.

It must be pointed out that it is not easy to be positive, especially when you are confronted by different life challenges and problems; as a matter of fact, it is easy to become overwhelmed by negative thinking even though you strive hard to stay positive. The key to success is to be fully *conscious* of what is going on in your mind, because all your negative actions and words are coming from your negative mind. In other words, stop your thinking mind as soon as you are aware that it begins to dwell on any negative thought. It is a general belief that the human mind can hold only one thought at a time. If this is true, then you have a choice: focusing on either the negative or the positive thought.

Develop the right attitude of *change*. Do not resist change because everything in life is forever changing whether you like it or not. You cannot stay exactly where you are, even though it may be your comfort zone. Life offers only few absolutes, and nothing is really set in stone. Any change in your life may be positive or negative. The key to positive living is to embrace *any* change, no matter what, as it comes along in your life.

Brain fitness

Exercise

Exercise boosts blood flow to your brain by promoting the development of more blood vessels and connections between brain cells. Exercise also increases the production of new brain cells for learning and remembering. Studies have repeatedly demonstrated that exercise can double or even triple the number of new cells, compared with the number in animals that do not exercise. If you wish to maintain your learning and remembering skills, exercise your body.

Regular endurance exercise, such as running, swimming, or biking, can also foster new brain cell growth and preserve existing brain cells. Build your physical endurance.

Strength training, such as lifting weights or using a resistance band, not only builds muscle and strengthens bone; but also boosts brain power, improves mood, enhances concentration, and increases decision-making skills. Build your physical strength.

Your flexibility gradually declines with age. Better flexibility means more energy, improved posture, and reduced risk of injury from falls. Build your flexibility with Tai chi, yoga, and stretching exercise.

Body balance diminishes progressively as you get older. Balance training is not just about avoiding falls. Better balance will improve your overall movement and your ability to do things better throughout your life. Build your body balance by standing on one foot or walking backward.

Diet

Eating foods high in saturated fats, like red meat, butter and dairy products, are associated with the development of degenerative diseases, such as heart disease, and Alzheimer's disease.

Fish is a great source of omega-3, the type of fatty acid your body cannot produce, and it is good for your brain. To get your omega-3, eat salmon, cod, haddock, tuna, halibut, and sardines. If you don't like fish, then eat plenty of walnuts, flaxseeds, and soybeans instead.

Leafy green vegetables, such as spinach, kale, broccoli, are loaded with nutrients good for the brain. Blueberries, raspberries and blackberries are packed with antioxidants that slow down aging in the brain.

Dark chocolate contains flavonoids, which are also strong antioxidants that potentially improve blood flow to the brain and reduce inflammation. Unsweetened cocoa powder is another excellent option.

Many herbs and spices, such as turmeric, cinnamon and ginger, are packed with antioxidants that may decrease harmful inflammation in the brain. Use these strong flavors in your cooking.

Whole grains, such as oats, barley, and quinoa, are rich in many of the B vitamins that work to reduce inflammation of the brain to prevent memory loss.

The protein and vitamins B, D and E in eggs and egg yolks may help improve memory. You can reap the benefits of these vitamins while keeping your cholesterol to a minimum by mixing whole eggs with egg whites to round out your omelet or scrambled eggs.

Music

According to some scientific research, music has the capacity and capability to change your neuron activity. Music therapists believe that the different sounds from different musical instruments have different impact on different body organs in the physical body. Scientists have used MP3 music and subliminal messages for practicing hypnosis to awaken the subconscious mind to improve memory, to enhance learning, to heal sleep problems, and to increase self-confidence, just to name a few possibilities. Music has to do with sound, which is one of the important sensory skills for maintaining good memory. In general, music listening and playing improves your concentration and brain power.

Brain reserve

Humans have "brain reserve," which helps the human brain adapt and respond to changes and resist damage. Your brain reserve begins to develop in childhood and gets stronger as you move through adulthood. People who continue to learn, embrace new activities, and develop new skills and interests are building and improving their brain reserve. Therefore, it is important to keep on learning new things to preserve the brain reserve.

Study

Get yourself educated. It can substantially increase your ability to fight off dementia. The same is true of working at a challenging job. So, go back to school, take classes, get a degree or an advanced degree. You are never too old to learn, and your brain will thank you in the long run.

Play

Do crossword puzzles, play chess, mahjong, card games, or online games. These activities can stimulate the brain. Playing electronic "brain games" may help you improve your reaction time and problem-solving ability. It is important to find one that you will want to continue to play.

The Healthy Mind Platter of Dr. Daniel Siegel

Dr. Daniel J. Siegel, professor of clinical psychiatry at the UCLA School of Medicine, has recommended *seven* daily essential mental activities to optimize brain health and creativity.

- Focusing on daily challenges helps your brain make some deep connections.
- Playing creatively and joyfully helps your brain make new connections.
- Connecting with nature and others daily helps your brain reinforce its relational circuitry.
- Moving aerobically helps your brain strengthen its brain cells.
- Reflecting internally, and focusing on sensations, feelings, thoughts, and images, help your brain integrate better.
- Relaxing without any mental focus helps your brain recharge.
- Sleeping restfully helps your brain consolidate and recover from the experiences of the day.

Consciousness of Spiritual Wellness

As opposed to materiality, spirituality is always invisible, immeasurable, but present and lasting. It is like the wind—it is invisible and yet palpable. It provides guidance, direction, and understanding to the mind. Spirituality takes the form of love, joy, and peace, and it is often expressed in human actions and behaviors. Materiality, on the other hand, is always visible, measurable, and transient. Humans need *both* spirituality and materiality: the former to understand the self, and the latter to understand the world and the universe around the self. Spirituality not only inspires the mind but also energizes the body—it is a body-mind-spirit connection necessary for the total wellness of an individual.

The pivotal role of spirituality

Your whole being is composed of the physical, the mental, and the spiritual. Your body—the physical—is controlled by your mind—the mental—which is supervised by your soul—the spiritual. Your spirituality oversees your whole being. Nothing transforms you as much as changing from a mundane to a spiritual attitude towards all your everyday problems.

Living in the physical world is challenging in itself. The challenges often turn themselves into toxins that infest the body as well as the mind. A mind is supposed to control the body, but an infested mind loses much of its control over the body, and thus letting the body do whatever it wants to do, and thus poisoning both the body and the mind. The role of the soul is to provide the mind with instructions and inspirations on how to take care of the body. But the toxins of the mind can also poison the soul, and thus not only stunting the growth of spirituality but also disconnecting the mind from its spiritual source.

There are often times when the mind is at a loss, confused, and helpless, and that is when the soul can be its inspiration and its awakening agent, provided the mind is willing to seek the help of the soul.

Letting go to attain wellness of the soul

Material attachment is a toxic thought that connects material things to the ego of an individual in the physical world. It is the reluctance of that individual to let go of material things that define who that individual thinks he or she is. Attachment to the ego-self and its related material things is the source of human woes, which impact the body and the mind, and ultimately contaminate the soul.

Bottom line: Let go of your ego-self (the gravitational center of attachment). At some point in your life, you have to let go of *all* your material things because they do not last, and neither do they define who you are. Letting go is the pathway to spiritual wellness.

In addition, emotional attachment is also a toxic thought that is a stumbling block to attaining spiritual wellness. For example, bitterness is a common and rampant toxic thought that batters the mind and bruises the soul. Bitterness cherishes anger, which often turns itself into rage, seeking revenge. Bitterness ultimately devastates the soul.

The bottom line: Do not justify your bitterness. The hurt never justifies the bitterness. Any desire for justice (making it personal) stains and blemishes the soul. Just let go of any attachment to bitterness.

> "Make every effort to live in peace with everyone and to be holy; without holiness no one will see the Lord. See to it no one falls short of the grace of God and that no bitter root grows up to cause trouble and defile many." (**Hebrews** 12:14-15)

Envy is another attachment that tarnishes the soul. Envy is tantamount to rejecting your own blessings because you are counting the blessings of others rather than yours. Envy is about comparing yourself with others. In life, it is important to believe in yourself. If you don't believe in yourself, how can you believe in your Creator? One of the obstacles to believing in yourself is comparing yourself with others. You are who you are; don't try to be someone else that you are not. Envy leads to craving: "wanting more and more" (greed) or "wanting more for less" (taking unfair advantage of others).

The bottom line: Be grateful for what you have; rejoice with those who have more. Let go of attachment to envy.

Fear is a debilitating toxic thought for the toxic soul. This toxic thought is manifested in many forms, such as fear of an outcome (disappointment), fear of loss (refusal to let go), fear of the future (lack of self-belief, or faith in the Creator), and fear of rejection (non-acceptance by others).

> **Jesus** said: "Can any one of you by worrying add a single hour to your life?" (**Matthew** 6:27)

> "Without faith it is impossible to please God." (**Hebrews** 11:6)

The bottom line: Let go of "what-ifs" from your mind; nobody knows the future anyway.

Strengthening spirituality

Spirituality is the wisdom to believe—believe in doing what is right and avoiding what is wrong. Many people are spiritual, even though they may not have a religion; they still believe that there is a Higher Being who is in control of the universe and what is happening around, such as the sun always comes out in the east. They are spiritual when they have a heart that feels for themselves as well as for others.

But *how* does one become more spiritual?

Your soul is your spirituality. Use your consciousness to strengthen your inherent spirituality: be aware of your body-mind-soul connection. Always seek spiritual wisdom.

> "Ask, and it will be given to you; seek, and you will find; knock, and it will be opened to you." (**Matthew** 7:7)

Simplify your life. Clear away all the physical clutters in your life as the first step towards freeing yourself from your material and mundane attachments. Material things do not define who you are. Once you have let go of the physical clutters in your living environment, you may then get to know more about yourself, especially your needs and values, instead of your desires and wants. Remember, needs and wants are not the same; your wants often create toxic desires and their accompanying toxic emotions, resulting in your attachments.

Learn to look within yourself for answers to your life problems: you will become more self-reliant and self-sufficient. Find your *inner voice*: what you love to do, and what touches your heart and your soul. Your inner self knows the *truth* when you hear it. Nobody knows you better than yourself—just as there is no better physician than yourself, who know what is best for your body. This intuitive wisdom is self-healing, which gives you a healthier body and mind to nourish your soul. Consciously improve your everyday attitudes and feelings, not just about yourself, but also towards others around you. Each and every moment in your day-to-day interactions with people may provide an opportunity for you to become more spiritual, if you consciously avail yourself of that opportunity to see miracles in your life. Using **Mother Teresa**'s example, begin by conveying warmth to someone who least expects it, and this generous gesture of compassion is a strong testament to your innate spirituality. It is your spiritual thinking that causes your personality and daily interactions with others to become an expression of your soul: your daily actions *speak* you mind. A healthy mind is full of spirituality.

Feed your mind with positive thoughts to avoid any distorted thinking that may disenfranchise your soul. Consistently replenish your soul with spiritual feelings, such as unconditional love, generosity, gratitude, and forgiveness, among others. Love melts your resistance to change for the better; without love, you simply continue to perpetuate that you resist, such as resisting to letting go. Generosity is freely giving your time and effort to others, as well as to yourself; it is paying others *forward* without any selfish interest or expectation. Gratitude will not make you compare your current state of health or wealth with that of others; gratitude is a great attitude in overcoming toxic thoughts of envy and greed that you may still attach to at the back of your mind. Forgiveness is a necessary requirement for health and healing of the mind and the soul; forgive yourself as well as others for all the mistakes done by you, or by others to you—mistakes are necessary for the learning process in life and the empowerment of the soul. Never look back in anger. Just let go of the past.

Spirituality, at a deeper level, means a desire to have a personal relationship with your Creator. Learn to pray. Prayers work by altering your brain chemistry. Like anti-depressant drugs, prayers can help you build up the feeling-good brain chemicals, such as serotonin. Prayers restore your hope, strength, and even health.

With the desire to believe, comes the awareness of your inner longings, as wells as your consciousness of an inner voice speaking to you—the growth and development of spirituality. Then, you must persist and persevere in your search and pursuit of spirituality, such as daily prayers and acts of right mindedness. Finally, further down the road, life crises and daily problems along your life journey may, surprisingly, further awaken you to your own innate spirituality.

To sum up, spirituality is the consciousness of your true self with the deep desire to become wholesome, connecting your body and your mind through your soul to form a divine relationship with the Creator. Spirituality, more importantly, is a deep longing to have a closer contact with the Creator to receive His Divine guidance in your everyday living, such that your mind may help your body in the miracle of living, thereby instrumental in letting go to let God take over.

If You Just Don't Die!

If you just don't die and go on living, life would be meaningless and even painful if you are unhappy and unhealthy: your body forever besieged by physical aches and pains; your mind often muddled in anxieties and sadness; and your soul now and then scourged by guilt and regret. Human happiness is the alignment of the body, the mind, and the soul; they have to be in balance and harmony before you can feel your happiness and life purpose. In other words, your mind, overseen and supervised by your soul, must also be able to control and manage your body, which must also be willing and compliant. Without this perfect alignment, there is no happiness.

FIVE

CONSCIOUSNESS OF LIVING

"Somebody should tell us, right at the start of our lives, that we are dying. Then we might live life to the limit, every minute of every day. Do it! I say. Whatever you want to do, do it now! There are only so many tomorrows." **Pope Paul VI**

Simplicity in Living

Consciousness of living a simple lifestyle is the key to happiness and longevity. In this day and age, living in this complex world of technology is not easy: The complexity of this world has taken a toll on the human mind, creating undue stress, as well as many emotional, mental, personal, and psychological attachments in the material world. For these reasons, profound human wisdom in living is essential to overcoming stress and letting go of all attachments. Simplicity is the first step towards detachment, which holds the key to unlocking the door to happiness. Live a simple lifestyle, deleting all the trimmings of life and living, as well as all the attachments that may have a negative impact on your mind.

Epicurus, the Greek philosopher, had this advice on how to lead a pleasant life: avoiding luxuries, and living simply. The explanation is that luxurious living may make you into a "needy" person whose happiness always depends on things that are impermanent and easily lost.

The late **Robert Kennedy** once said: "Sometimes I think that the only people in this country who worry more about money than the poor are the very wealthy. They worry about losing it, they worry about how it is invested, they worry about the effect it's going to have. And as the zeroes increase, the dilemmas get bigger."

Can you live a simple lifestyle to help you let go of all the trimmings of life?

When you were in your younger days, you might have had many attachments to life that define who you were, such as the car you were driving, the designer dress you were wearing, or anything that defined your social status. Can you, at this point in your life, let go of all these attachments and just lead a simple life?

A classic example is **Ann Russell Miller**, a celebrated socialite from San Francisco, also known as **Sister Mary Joseph**, She, who had ten children and nineteen grand-children, had grown up in luxury and privilege, and had been living a life of incredible wealth. Instead of shopping at Saks Fifth Avenue, and decorating herself with jewelry from Tiffany, she suddenly decided to give up everything, and became a nun devoted to living in poverty for the rest of her life. That unbelievable event happened more than two decades ago, and was then widely reported in the media across the country. Why did she make such a drastic and incredible change in her life? She said she had a calling, a true vocation that was hard to understand for the general public, even for the close members of her family.

With less focus on your attachments to the material world, your heart will be more on your spirituality.

> "For where your treasure is, there your heart will be also." (**Matthew** 6:21)

With spirituality, you may be more willing to let go of everything you hold on to in your life.

> "The Spirit is just like water flowing to all things.
> Its true nature is to give life indiscriminately to all.
> It flows to low places, where people reject and despise.
> It flows like a river, nurturing everything and everyone on its way.
> Its final stop is the ocean, which is its very origin.
>
> Living by the Spirit, we choose a simple and humble lifestyle.
> We meditate to enhance our spirituality.
> We love our neighbors as ourselves.
> We express compassion to all.
>
> We speak with truth and sincerity.
> We live in the present moment.
> We take action only when necessary.
>
> Without much ado or over-doing, we trust the guidance of the Spirit.

In this manner, life flows like water, fulfilling itself and also everything naturally."
(Lao Tzu, *Tao Te Ching*, chapter 8)

Living in simplicity is living a humble life, which is emptying your toxic cravings and attachments.

"All of us also lived among them at one time, gratifying the cravings of our flesh and following its desires and thoughts. Like the rest, we were by nature deserving of wrath."
(**Ephesians** 2:3)

Attachments create your ego-self that not only separates you from others but also gives you your pride, instead of humility.

"Focusing on status gives us pride, and not humility.
Hoarding worldly riches deprives us of heavenly assets.

An empty mind with no craving and no expectation helps us let go of everything.
Being in the world and not of the world, we attain heavenly grace."
(Lao Tzu, *Tao Te Ching*, chapter 2)

But with humility, we may see who we really are, not what we wish we were, and what we really need, not what we want. Humility is self-enlightening.

"Ever humble, we see the mysteries of all things created.
Ever proud, we see only the manifestations of

all things created.

Only the mysteries, and not the manifestations,
show us the Way to true wisdom."
(Lao Tzu, *Tao Te Ching*, chapter 1)

Live a simple life, especially as you continue to age, and you just don't die!

Living in the Present

Sister Mary Joseph would not have looked back to the past, to the luxurious life of **Ann Russell Miller**; instead, she would continue to live in the present, the simple life she had chosen.

Simplicity gives your clarity of thinking to see the wisdom of living in the present: the past was gone; the future is yet to come, and only the present is real—a gift from the Creator, and that is why it is called "present."

"Simplicity is clarity.
It is a blessing to learn from those
with humble simplicity.

Those with an empty mind
will learn to find the Way.

The Way reveals the secrets of the universe:
the mysteries of the realm of creation;
the manifestations of all things created.
The essence of the Way is to show us
how to live in fullness and return to our origin."
(Lao Tzu, *Tao Te Ching*, chapter 65)

Clarity of thinking may let you have the true human wisdom to know your true nature, thereby ending your craving and hence your self-imposed suffering.

> "Our greatest suffering comes from
> not knowing who we are, or to whom we belong."
> (Lao Tzu, *Tao Te Ching*, chapter 46)

In the present moment, with clarity of mind, you may begin to see the ultimate truths of the self, others, as well as everything around you. More importantly, you may see your past follies in identifying yourself with your thoughts that have created your ego-self, your present futile efforts in striving to protect your ego-self, and your future futilities in expecting that your ego-self will all its attachments will continue to exist in the days to come.

Living in the present is an awakening to the realities of all things. It may afford you an opportunity to look more *objectively* at any given situation, allowing your mind to think more clearly, to separate the truths from the self-deceptions that might have been created in your subconscious minds all along.

> "Living in the present moment,
> we see all things that we must do.
> Without complaint and resistance, we do them accordingly.
> Without seeking control and recognition,
> we simplify what we do, however complicated they may be.
> Trusting in the Creator, we always under-do and never over-do."
> (Lao Tzu, *Tao Te Ching*, chapter 30)

72

Living in the present is mindfulness of what is happening to you and around you, enabling you to understand the impermanence of all things, and hence the need to let go of all attachments that prevent from living a contented life.

> "Living in the present moment,
> we find natural contentment.
> We do not seek a faster lifestyle,
> or a better place to be.
> We need the essentials of life,
> not its extra trimmings.
>
> Living in the present moment,
> we focus on the experience of the moment.
> Thus, we enjoy every aspect of simple living,
> and find contentment in everyone and
> everything.
>
> Living in contentment,
> we grow old and die,
> feeling contented."
> (Lao Tzu, *Tao Te Ching*, chapter 80)

Focusing on the present moment liberates you from projecting your desires into the future as expectations that necessitate your over-doing to guarantee their fulfillment.

> "Therefore, we focus on the present moment,
> doing what needs to be done,
> without straining and stressing.
>
> To end our suffering,
> we focus on the present moment,

instead of our expected result.
So, we follow the natural laws of things."
(Lao Tzu, *Tao Te Ching*, chapter 63)

Most importantly, living in the present is synonymous with letting go of control: controlling the future based on assumptions of the past. Control is basic human instinct. Humans are inherently controlling. Out of fear and insecurity, our ancestors living as early as in the Stone Age strove to control their environment in order to survive, developing their fight-or-flight instinct. Most of us are controlling to a certain extent. We, as parents, control our children's destinies by striving to steer them clear of the wrong pathways we had previously treaded ourselves. Our culture tells us that we should be in control of everything around us at all times, including our futures and destinies. Living in the present may help you let go of controlling because you never know what would happen tomorrow because your Creator is in control of everything in your life.

> "So do not worry, saying, 'What shall we eat?' or 'What shall we drink?' or 'What shall we wear?' For the pagans run after all these things, and your heavenly Father knows that you need them. But seek first his kingdom and his righteousness, and all these things will be given to you as well. Therefore do not worry about tomorrow, for tomorrow will worry about itself. Each day has enough trouble of its own."
> (**Matthew** 6:31-34)

Letting go of control may further enlighten you to understand that everything follows a natural cycle.

Following the Natural Cycle

Everything in life must follow a natural cycle, whether we like it or not, and we must be patient and obedient.

> "That which shrinks
> Must first expand.
> That which fails,
> Must first be strong.
> That which is cast down
> Must first be raised.
> Before receiving, there must be giving.
> This is called perception of the nature of
> things.
> Soft and weak overcome hard and strong."
> (Lao Tzu, *Tao Te Ching*, chapter 36)

Spontaneity is the essence of the natural cycle. What goes up must eventually come down; life only begets death; day is always followed by night—they are just like the cycle of the four seasons.

> "Allowing things to come and go,
> following their natural laws,
> we gain everything.
> Straining and striving,
> we lose everything."
> (Lao Tzu, *Tao Te Ching*, chapter 48)

Intuition of spontaneity is an understanding of the impermanence of all things: nothing lasts no matter how hard we strive to keep them permanent, and everything remains only with that present moment, and it never lasts. Gaining that understanding is wisdom of the mind to let go of everything in life.

> "Strong winds come and go.
> So do torrential rains.
> Even heaven and earth cannot make them last
> forever.
> Why then so much concern over what to say,
> or what to do?
> Living is but an expression of the life given by
> the Creator.
> Our true nature is a reflection of that
> expression."
> (Lao Tzu, *Tao Te Ching*, chapter 23)

Following the natural cycle of all things, we must be patient with and obedient to what the Creator has planned for us:

> "Trusting in the Creator, we see the comings
> and goings of things,
> but without straining and striving to control
> them."
> (Lao Tzu, *Tao Te Ching*, chapter 29)

If You Just Don't Die

If you just don't die and continue with your life, you will have to learn how to live in the now, because you never know if tomorrow will ever come again. In addition, you will have to let go of all the trimmings of life—your material possessions, as well as your past and your memories of the past, because some day you might not even have any memory left to remember them.

SIX

CONSCIOUSNESS OF CHANGES AND CHALLENGES

"Progress is impossible without change, and those who cannot change their minds cannot change anything." **George Bernard Shaw**

"When we meet real tragedy in life, we can react in two ways—either by losing hope and falling into self-destructive habits, or by using the challenge to find our inner strength. " Dalai Lama

Everything in this world we are living in is changing every moment. Change is constant and continuous. Change is inevitable. Change can be positive or negative. No matter what, we have only three options: deny the change; accept and embrace it, or change ourselves to adapt to the change.

The first option—denying the change—is self-delusive. Besides, living a static life without any change could be boring and meaningless.

The second option—accepting and embracing the

change—is sometimes necessary because the change is inevitable and irreversible, such as the change caused by death and bereavement.

The third option—changing the self to adapt to the change—is often the outcome of the second option.

Negative Changes

There are many changes in life that occur due to aging, and they are inevitable, although these changes can be slowed down.

Vision deterioration

Your vision, the most important asset in your life, changes throughout your life journey. The human eye is not just a mechanical tool for vision; it is one of the body's most important organs. Because they are hardwired into your brain, your eyes are an extension of your brain: they give you your uniquely individual perception and vision of the outside world, as well as a reflection of how and what you think.

Your eyesight is the most important of your five senses. Because it affects your perception, attitude, behavior, and personality; it is instrumental in creating your own world, especially if you just don't die. Your vision also affects your health because your eyes are inter-connected with many of your body organ, such as your brain (which controls how you see), your heart (which pumps blood and transports oxygen to your eyes), and your liver (which supplies nutrients to your eyes). Therefore, healthy vision requires a healthy mind and a healthy body. Vision fitness involves balancing what you see and what you think.

But, unfortunately, your vision deteriorates with gradual decline in health in both your body and mind as you add more years to your life.

Coping with vision problems

Poor vision is lack of clarity when seeing near or far away objects, or with insufficient light. Poor vision is mainly caused by mental stress and eye muscle strain.

Total mind and body relaxation

The eye conditions are constantly changing such that they can be adversely affected by any emotional or mental stress, resulting in eyestrain that can cause vision blur. By the same token, you can significantly improve your vision if you relax your eyes completely through total body-mind relaxation. But it is almost impossible to relax just your eyes, while the rest of your body remains tense and stressed. Total relaxation begins with the mind first, and then the rest of the body, including the eye. Use your mind to relax your body, and then your eyes. The best way to achieve total body-mind relaxation is by meditation.

Total eye relaxation

Your eyes are active throughout your waking hours. As a result, they are constantly in strain and stress. Your eyes simply do not know how to relax, unless they receive direct instructions from your conscious mind, or when they are in total darkness.

Correcting bad vision habits

Bad vision habits occur when you unconsciously strain and stress your eyes by fixating or staring (healthy eyes are constantly "shifting" from one detail to another); by seeing with unbalanced vision (that is, one eye is much stronger than the other one, for example, lazy eye), that is, using only the central vision of your eyes to see, while neglecting their peripheral vision, and thus leading to restricted vision field (healthy eyes see with *both* central vision and peripheral vision); and by squinting your eyes from "excess" light (healthy eyes easily adapt and adjust to excess or insufficiency of light).

Use your mind to consciously correct your bad vision habits by doing the following consciously:

- Improve your *eye shifting*: train your mind to edge or trace the outline of any visual object with your eyes. Form this good vision habit to avoid "staring" or "fixation" of your eyes. For example, while waiting for the bus, train your eyes to trace the outline of buildings in the distance.

- Enhance your *eye balancing:* wear an eye-patch (obtainable at your local pharmacy) over your stronger eye in order to strengthen your weaker eye.

- Promote better *periphery vision* in your eyes: use different-size eye-patches to partially cover your eyes for 20 minutes in order to enhance your peripheral vision. After the exercise, you will feel that your vision has "expanded" temporarily.

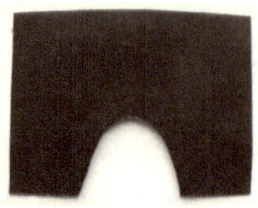

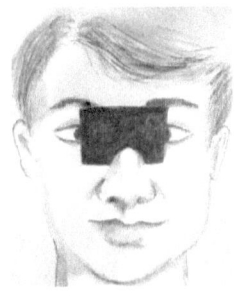

- Minimize *squinting* of your eyes: avoid wearing sunglasses as much as possible to let your eyes get accustomed to stronger light.

With good vision habits, your eyes will "naturally observe" or "notice" what is around; your eyes will never "strain" to see *everything*; your eyes will relax and rest even when it is "looking."

Self-massage eye exercise

Gently and slowly massage your eyes for total relaxation to increase blood circulation, to create a sense of ease about seeing, as well as to enhance the awareness of your eyes for better vision.

- Breathe deeply and slowly.
- Rub both hands to generate warmth.
- Massage your jaw with your hands moving in small circles, from your chin outward along your jawbone up to the front of and behind your ears.
- Then slowly move your hands over the bridge of your nose, and massage outward along your cheekbones until you reach your temples and your ears.

- Then, starting from the bridge of your nose, massage along your eyebrows, moving above, below, and along the brow. Use your thumbs to press against the grooves slightly below your eyebrow ridge close to the bridge of your nose.
- Gently squeeze your eyeball with your fingers.
- Finally, use long, firm, strokes to massage your forehead from the left to the right, and then from the right to the left.

Throughout your facial and eye self-massage, look for sore spots, especially in the eyebrow area. Massage them with slightly harder and stronger circular movements.

Rubbing-the-eye-and-eyelid exercise

- Apply and press the heel of your left palm and the heel of your right palm against your left eye and right eye, respectively.
- With gentle pressure, rub them with a twisting movement, your left eye with your left palm and your right eye with your right palm.
- Meanwhile, contract and relax your eyelid muscles.

Open-and-squeeze eye exercise

This ancient Chinese exercise, developed by Taoists monks thousands of years ago, increases blood circulation to your eyes, prevents your watery eyes, and alkalizes your eyes to detoxify your liver. This exercise also removes your eye strain and soothes your eye-muscle tension.

- Inhale slowly, while squeezing your eyes tightly for 10 seconds.
- Then, slowly exhale your breath, making the *sh-h-h-h-h-h* sound, while opening your eyes wide.
- Repeat as many times and as often as required to cleanse your eyes and your liver.

Eye-stretching exercise

Master this eye-muscle stretching exercise to relieve your eye tension and maintain your eye relaxation.

- Sit comfortably, taking a few deep breaths.
- Stretch your eyes upward as far as they can go without straining them.
- Hold your breath. Stretch your eyes downward as you exhale.
- Repeat this up-and-down movement of your eyes a few times.
- Stretch your eyes by moving them around in circles but without straining them, as you breathe in and breathe out.

Eye-palming exercise

This unique eye-relaxation exercise uses your healing hands to direct energy to your eyes, as well as to rest your optic nerve, and relax your entire nervous system.

- Sit comfortably with your elbows resting on a table in front of you—preferably in a totally darkened room. Rub your palms together to generate some heat and warmth.

- Place your palms over your eyes, without touching them, while resting them on the boney ridge and surrounding your eyes with the heels of your hands on your cheekbones. Your eyes should be *gently* but not *firmly* closed.
- Relax your mind, and breathe deeply through your nose, not your mouth. The slower your breathing is, the more relaxed your mind becomes.
- Feel your abdomen and back expand and contract as you inhale and exhale, respectively.
- Visualize complete darkness to further relax your mind.
- Feel your neck and shoulders expand and contract as your deep and slow breathing continues.
- Visualize every part of your body—hands, fingers, toes, knees, and thighs—expand and contract with your inhalation and exhalation.

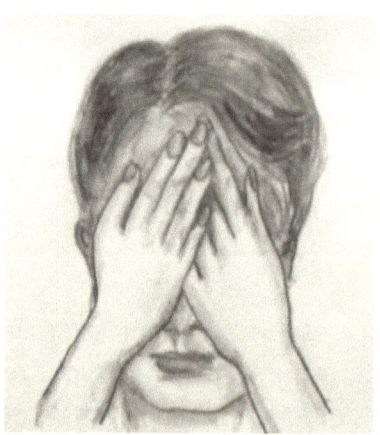

Practice eye-palming exercise as often as you feel fatigue in your eyes. A 10-minute session will work wonders to relax your eyes. You can practice it during commercial breaks on the television, or take regular breaks from your computer. This is the best eye-relaxation exercise.

Blinking exercise

If you do not blink frequently enough, you will not be able to see well. It is just that simple. Blinking has many vision benefits: it overcomes the harmful habit of staring; it relaxes the eye; it cleanses and massages the eye; it improves nearsightedness.

Learn how to blink, not squint. The former relaxes the eye, while the latter stresses the eye because it uses undue force to close and open the eye. Practice the following blinking exercise to make blinking second nature to you:

- Breathe deeply.
- Close and open your eyes. The blink has to be soft, not hard, and it must be complete. Imagine using your eyelashes to cause your eyes to close and open. Practice this several times until you master it. You may even have to count while you blink to make sure you do not blink too fast.
- Close your right eye, and cover it with your right hand.
- Blink your left eye. If the blink is soft, and not forced, your right hand over your right eye will *not* feel any movement. It is important that your blinking has to be soft and effortless.
- Repeat the process with the other eye.

Always remember to blink several times *before* you look at something in *both* close vision and distant vision.

Eye-accommodation exercise

Enhance and strengthen the accommodation of your

eyes. Due to aging, your accommodative eye muscles might have weakened and deteriorated due to lack of use. Follow the ancient Hindu yogis technique to strengthen your accommodative eye muscles so that you can see in the distance and also at close point. More importantly, they enable your eyes to easily change and shift their focus through improving the flexibility of your accommodative eye muscles.

- Write a few big black letters on a 2" x 3" card. Hold it at eye level and at arm's length away. Make sure you can see the letters clearly.
- Then, look at a distant object and see it clearly.
- Begin, one eye at a time, looking at the black letters at close distance, and then looking at a distant object, and then with both eyes.
- As your vision improves, move the card closer to you.

Light-adjusting exercise

Given that light is essential to good vision, it is important that you train your eyes to adjust comfortably to light, otherwise you may have a tendency to squint your eyes when the light is too bright or too dim.

Eye sunning exercise helps your eyes adjust to the change in the intensity of light. Sunning the eye is an exercise that utilizes the energy from the sun for healing your eye and improving your vision. The healing power of sunlight should come into the eye at a diagonal angle, and the sunlight should not be strong (that is, early in the morning, before 9 -10 a.m. and late in afternoon, after 5 - 6 p.m.)

- Sit or stand outdoors, your body facing the sun. You can also sit or stand at an open window, but do not let the sunlight come through glass (it has to be direct, not filtered, sunlight).
- Close your eyes; do not wear sunglasses. Let the sun bathe your eyes.
- Now, move your head slowly but constantly from side to side.
- Breathe in and out deeply and slowly. Relax your head, shoulders, and eyes, while continuing your body motion.
- Turn your back to the sun, and briefly palm your eyes for a few minutes during which you visualize blackness in your mind's eye.
- Return to the original position, and resume your eye sunning.
- Alternate between sunning and palming your eyes. You will soon notice that during sunning, the color seems brighter, while the blackness seems blacker during palming.
- Practice this for 10 to 20 minutes a day, if the weather permits.

Regular eye exercise is an integral part of your vision improvement. There are many eye exercises for vision improvement. Do as many as you can. Now in your golden years, you should be able to find more time to exercise your eyes to compensate for your loss of vision over the years. Eye exercises, however, do not produce immediate results, so you must be consistent and persistent in this endeavor to reap all the benefits of eye exercises. You must believe that those eye exercises can help your vision improvement to compensate for your vision loss.

Memory decline

The brain, as one of the most important body organs as well as the control center of your life and well-being, undergoes changes, resulting in memory decline. The degree of decline varies in individuals due to their differences in lifestyle and their genetic makeup. Memory loss is an impediment, but do not let it be your stumbling block in the rest of your life journey.

<u>Senior moments</u>

The human mind declines and memories start to wane after the age of 30 or so. As many people hit middle age, they often start to notice that their memory and mental clarity are not what they used to be. They suddenly cannot remember where they put their keys or eyeglasses just a moment ago, or an old acquaintance's name or even the name of an old band they used to love. As the brain fades, they euphemistically refer to these occurrences as "senior moments." Senior moments are becoming increasingly annoying and even frustrating as you continue in your aging process.

Have you, too, experienced your senior moments?

Frailty of memory may be due to many factors, including brain damage, alcohol and nicotine use, constipation, and dehydration (common among seniors due to their reduced consumption of water for fear of incontinence), depression, and pharmaceutical drugs (especially those anesthetic agents, benzodiazepines, and among others).

The storage of information in the brain hinges on *consciousness*. First of all, you must be fully conscious of its importance *before* you will decide to store it. If you think it is *really* important, then you must put it away in a safe place where you can easily retrieve it later. Finally, when you want to retrieve it, you must know or remember *where* to look for it. It is all about *consciousness*.

In the scenario of not knowing where you have put your keys or eyeglasses, first and foremost, you must make an immediate *deliberate* mental note that you will need your keys or eyeglasses as soon as you take them off; then, be *conscious* of the *place* where you put them, for example, right next to your cell phone or in front of the TV; when you need to find them, you can readily *recall* the place where you put them.

Of course, another option is to put your keys or eyeglasses in an assigned place, where you can always find them, but that will not help you *remember* where you put them. In addition, it may not always be possible to put them in the same place all the time. The bottom line: learn to be *conscious* of any new information you want to retrieve later, and make a deliberate effort to *remember* where you store that information. You must always train your mind for better memory. Just practice this consciousness not just for your keys or eyeglasses but for all other things. With more practice, you will soon find that your memory has significantly improved, instead of having deteriorated further due to lack of use!

Managing memory-loss problems

Memory-loss problems may often interfere with your daily living throughout the rest of your life. The good news is that numerous conditions associated with memory impairment are treatable and even reversible, especially when the conditions causing the delirium are successfully addressed, such as deficiency in vitamin B_{12}, autoimmune diseases, and depression. However, when these memory-loss conditions remain untreated for more than six months to a year, clinical experience has suggested that the prognosis for full recovery of memory function may become slim and the damage to mental health may be even permanent and irreversible.

To manage your memory-loss problems, you may try mnemonic aids (use of lists and reminders) and self-cuing. Use visual cues and mental associations to "jog" your memory.

Learn to process new information step by step, and one step at a time, to allow yourself more time to get the hang of it.

Avoid prescription drugs wherever possible. Over-the-counter drugs, such as sleeping pills, and antihistamines, such as *Benadryl* and *Tylenol PM*, contain dangerous chemicals, which may cause memory loss or decline. Anti-anxiety medications and antidepressants may also have adverse side effects on the brain. Avoid them as much as possible.

Go off the beaten track to break your old habits from time to time in order to stimulate your brain cells. According to **Dr. Randolph B. Schiffer**, Director of the Cleveland Clinic Lou Ruvo Center for Brain Health, occasionally going off the beaten track is "good for the soul." So, every now and then, do something out of the ordinary just to stimulate your brain.

Engage in challenging endeavors, such as crossword puzzles, adult learning, or learning a musical instrument.

Reduce stress, which interferes with concentration and staying focused. Anxiety dampens your mental ability, especially your memory skills to recall stored information.

Learn to use the Chinese Tai Chi breathing to inhale memories and exhale worries. Tai Chi not only de-stresses you but also enhances your mental alertness, in particular, your memory power. Change the incorrect way you breathe to avoid breathing difficulties, which are common among the elderly. Learn the correct way to breathe for total relaxation.

Use meditation to relax your body and mind for better memory enhancement.

Apply the principle of "present-mindedness" to avoid absent-mindedness and to focus on the present moment. You just need to be aware of an action *while* it is taking place, and not *after* it has already taken place, because it will be too late by then. This "present awareness" can be applied to almost anything you do in your daily life. What you need is to practice consciousness and concentration.

Of course, the best and most effective way to manage your memory is to *use* it, instead of relying on cues or reminders.

<u>Sharpening memory</u>

You have a great body, but you also need a great mind to go along with it. Therefore, exercise your cognitive faculties as you continue to age. Aging is normally associated with drawbacks in gathering and processing information, as well as language functioning. However, as you age, you may still retain your full or nearly full mental capacity, including your cognitive functions. In other words, in spite of your aging, *normal* mental health should enable you to learn new things, to remember and retain the new information acquired, to communicate with others, and to solve simple everyday problems. Given that your brain is the most important piece of real estate that you own, you need to keep it mentally and physically active in order to maintain its value.

Writing

Writing is a complex mental task. It sharpens the mind:

you have to think, to choose the right word, to connect words to make sense, and to organize sentences into paragraphs. You do not have to write *well* in order to write. You do not need to have a lot of ideas *before* you can write. If you are diligent at writing, ideas will come to you spontaneously. If you feel inadequacy in writing, begin writing a diary or a journal—that should make you feel more at ease because nobody is going to read it anyway. Write a letter or send an email to keep in touch with your friends. Writing regularly sharpens your memory. Write a blog or even a book.

Reading

Reading improves the many functions of the brain. It is a well-recognized brain booster. Read regularly. Also, take a meaningful break every half hour or so and try to *recall* what you have just read to keep your memory fresh and strong. Recalling is good practice of memory skills. According to **Charles A. Weaver III**, professor of psychology and neuroscience, "Reading increases the number of active cells in your brain, and the more active cells you have, the more connections you have between neurons, the active cells of the nervous system."

De-cluttering

The fewer clutters you have, the more organized you become, and the less stressful life is to you. Get rid of all the physical clutters in your home: this reduces stress and frustration when looking for things. Having fewer physical clutters means fewer mental clutters in your mind, so you can remember the things that are *really* important for you. Letting go of physical clutters is the first step in removing mental and spiritual clutters.

Sleeping

The process of storing memories continues even while you sleep. It is in this deepest dream state, known as Rapid Eye Movement (REM) sleep, that you store your memories. To sharpen your memory, you need to sleep well and to maintain a healthy sleep routine at all times.

Gardening

Sharpen your brain power with your green thumbs. Gardening is a good exercise for your body and mind: you need to know the plant names, their different growth characteristics, the soil conditions, and abstract spatial thinking. They all help you exercise your brain. Don't employ a landscaper to do your garden, do it yourself and save your money too!

Remembering what you want to remember.

Develop a photographic memory at any age, even as you step into seniority.

Memory has everything to do with *consciousness* and *mental associations*. You must be able to *associate* the information and input it in your brain, so that you can retrieve the information later. To facilitate the mental processing of the information, you need to do the following:

Concentration

Try not to do too many things too quickly at the same time. This not only creates time-stress but also disorients the mind. Forget about multi-tasking; most probably, by now, you have passed that age!

Visualization

Visualize the information in your mind's eye, which is essentially the process of *remembering*. Seeing is believing, and a picture is worth a thousand words. If you can vividly visualize something in your mind's eye, your memory of that becomes more vivid, and that memory will be retained much longer.

Creativity and imagination

Being creative and imaginative is an indispensable asset in good memory. The explanation is that with a creative mind, you can come up with mental associations that are totally outrageous and therefore unforgettable. The more absurd your mental associations are, the longer they will stick in your memory. You can learn to become more creative and imaginative through more practice. If you can think of something extraordinary, you can create out-of-the-ordinary mental associations that you will not easily forget. For example, when you are introduced to someone by the name of "Dustin", you can create the image of a *dustbin*, and associate the features of that person with a dustbin. The more ridiculous that image is, the more you will remember that person's name.

Repetition

Give the information a sound so that you can *hear* it as well as *see* it. Repeat the information as much as possible. For example, if you are introduced to a person, repeat the name of that person several times to register it in your brain.

However, the process of repeating and remembering may not be as simple and straightforward as you wish: there may be obstacles to hindering the process. These obstacles may include distraction, lack of focus, inadequate motivation, and a stressful environment.

Compartmentalization

Finally, you need to store the information in an organized and systematic way in a mental folder in your memory. The human mind has a great capacity for storage of information. In fact, you have probably used up only about ten percent of brain storage space available. To help you remember all types of information as well as to retrieve all the stored information, you need to think *logically* and *categorize* systematically the information in your mind's eye. The brain is like a file cabinet, where you put many different types of information according to different categories or headings.

Physical frailty

One of the changes in the human body is the reduction of physical strength that leads to physical frailty due to aging. Frailty may often lead to falls, physical disability, ultimate immobility, and even death.

Preventing frailty

In the psychological area, avoid *depression*, which is common as you advance in age. In the cognitive area, defer *dementia*. In the physical realm, maintain *mobility* for as long as you can; keep your sensory organs sharp and functional, such as vision and hearing. In the social domain, set up *social connections*, get support from friends and groups, and do volunteer work. In short, activities may keep your frailty at bay.

Falling and immobility

Falling is the No.1 debilitating factor in aging and frailty because it creates *fear* among the elderly, instrumental in immobilizing them into a mental and physical state of inertia, which often brings about rapid decline in the mental faculty. Over-concern or fear of falling may also result in the repercussion of physical inactivity, and thus leading to immobility in the elderly.

Aging neither imposes certain limitations on your physical body, nor does it necessarily make you fall. You fall because you are immobile. Being physically active and maintaining good posture as well as body balance hold the key to preventing falls. Maintain your mobility through activities and good posture and body balance.

Causes of falling

There are many factors that may cause you to fall. Falling is due to both external and internal conditions.

Some of the external conditions are inadequate lighting and too many scattered objects in the environment. Improve the environment by de-cluttering and providing sufficient lighting. The internal conditions may include body imbalance caused by circulatory problems, diseases, such as arthritis and osteoporosis, medications, such as sedatives, mental problems due to confusion and dementia, muscular weakness, and poor vision. All of these health-related conditions could make you become either more inactive out of fear of falling, or more prone to falling. Therefore, to prevent falling, you need to address all those issues that predispose you to the high risks of falling.

Preventing falls

Develop your mental concentration, which plays a pivotal role in preventing falls. Enhance your consciousness through daily meditation, complemented by breathing exercise. Sharpen your mental awareness of what is happening around you.

Fear is not anti-aging. As a matter of fact, fear is the No.1 obstacle in practicing and repeating certain movements on a regular basis aimed at enhancing your body balance to improve your flexibility for both physical and emotional well-being. Over-caution constricts your muscles, making them more tense and inflexible, and thus further impairing your body balance system. The key to overcoming fear is not to avoid any situation that might cause you to fall; instead, move around to avoid it, and thereby preventing falls. Movement, activity, and exercise promote and enhance your mental, emotional, and social well-being. As you continue to age, it is important to make what seems impossible become fun and possible to you.

Maintaining body balance

Find your own *focal point* by focusing your eyes on an object. Practice your body balance by slightly raising one foot, either right or left, in the following positions:

- Both hands on your hips
- Both hands at your sides
- Both hands outstretched sideways
- Both hands raised above your head in a "V" position

Stretching

Stretching has substantial health benefits: it increases your mobility range, your muscle flexibility, your energy level, your blood circulation, and your protection against injury should you happen to fall. Stretch your limbs before you get out of bed every morning.

Strengthening legs for balance, equilibrium, and mobility

- Sit on a chair, and relax, with feet apart, and hands on your sides.
- Stand up a little, with legs bent, and hands on your sides, and HOLD at a count of five.
- Next, stand up a little more, with legs still slightly bent, and hands on your sides, and HOLD at a count of five.
- Now, stand up straight and tall, and HOLD at a count of five.
- Reverse and repeat the process until you sit down on the chair.

Strengthening ankles and feet for balance and flexibility

- Stand tall with your feet slightly apart.
- Slowly raise both heels from the floor, and HOLD for a count of five.
- Slowly lower both heels, and relax.
- Repeat five to ten times.

Enhancing body balance and flexibility

- Stand tall, your feet slightly apart, with your arms stretched out sideways for body balance.
- Slowly bend your right knee, and cross your right foot in front of and to the outside of your left foot, touching your right toes to the floor.
- With your right knee still bent, slowly and gently SWING your right leg from the front position to behind your left leg, touching your right toes to the floor. Use your stretched out arms to balance if necessary.
- Repeat the activity using your left foot.

It is important to exercise in order to create constant mobility to enhance eye-hand-foot coordination, to promote motor skills to reduce reaction time, to heighten spatial awareness, to improve posture and poise, and to increase mental capability with more oxygen supply from your bloodstream. Strengthen some of your inactive muscles that may cause body imbalance, contributing to falling. By the time you are in your senior years, you may have lost 20 to 40 percent of your muscles—and, along with it, their strength. Scientists have discovered that a major reason you lose muscle is that you have stopped doing everyday activities that use those inactive muscles, and not just because you are growing older.

According to the American Heart Association, keeping your muscles inactive for long periods of time hurts your health. Move around and walk even when you are doing your normal daily routine, such as talking on the phone; get up and walk about, instead of switching TV channels during the commercial breaks; getting into the habit of parking further away from your destination. Always avoid a sedentary lifestyle that promotes inactive muscles. Always lead a life full of spirit and vigor in your senior years to increase muscle strength and flexibility.

No matter how careful you are, there will be times when an accidental fall may happen to you. However, if your body remains loose and flexible, your injury may be reduced to a minimum. The more fit your feet and legs are, the more resistant you will be to falls. Frequent and repeated falls may ultimately impair your long-term mobility, resulting in rapid health decline as you continue to age. Therefore, do everything you can to maintain your mobility, which may add many more years to your life.

Health degeneration

Another major change in the human body is the onset of disease. No matter how well you take care of your health through diet and exercise, disease may be unavoidable. However, early detection of disease signs and symptoms may go a long way to eradicating it before causing irreparable damage.

Consciousness of disease signs and symptoms

Fatigue

Fatigue is often an initial sign of a disease. Chronic fatigue is a complex and debilitating disorder that is not alleviated by bed rest. Fatigue is an indication of disharmony between the body and the mind. Sharpen your mental awareness and concentration to relieve your body of tension and your mind of compulsive thoughts.

Weight loss

A sudden and unexplained weight loss is also a symptom

of the development of an imminent disease, such as cancer, diabetes, depression, liver disease, or even an overactive thyroid. Be conscious of an unintentional loss of up to 10 percent of your body weight within a few months.

Difficulty in breathing

Breathlessness, such as gasping for air or wheezing, can be a tale-telling sign of asthma, a blood clot, bronchitis, obstructive pulmonary disease, pneumonia, as well as other heart and lung diseases. Of course, an episode of panic attack may also result in breathlessness.

Changes in bowels

Bloody, black, or tarry-colored stools are often signs of diarrhea or constipation, while unexplained urges to have a bowel movement may signal a bacterial infection, colon cancer, or irritable bowel syndrome (IBS), a disorder that often leads to abdominal pain and cramping.

Physical pain

Pain is often a signal sent by the brain that there is a problem somewhere within the body. Pain is more of a symptom than a disease in itself. Arthritis, rheumatism, and degenerating spinal discs can cause health problems other than just inducing pain. Pain does not necessarily originate from the source of the problem; for example, your spinal problem may give you a headache.

Consciousness of the body's nine openings

According to ancient Chinese medicine, the human body

has nine openings: the body, like a house, has seven windows, a front door, and a back door. The seven windows are the five sensing openings: two eyes, two ears, two nostrils, and the mouth; the front door is the genital, and the back door is the anus. These openings are the thresholds through which the body interacts with the outside world, and through which energy, information, and matter from the outside world are assimilated by the body.

The back door

The colon is the most important opening to manage in the physical body. Like the body's sewage system, it is responsible for the absence or presence of all the toxins in the body. It affects the brain and the nervous system (mental health), the heart, the lungs, and the whole body system.

Internal cleansing is the key to a healthy colon. It is detoxification, involving dislodging body toxins and waste products from within and between cells and joints, and then transporting these wastes from the body for disease prevention and treatment, for joint and muscle flexibility, weight loss and weight management, softening blood vessels and reducing blood pressure, as well as clean and clear skin.

Fasting is voluntary abstinence from foods and drinks, except water, for an extended period. Fasting is internal cleansing and rejuvenation—one of the most efficient ways to detoxify the body of toxins. Fasting is to recovery, as sleep is to recuperation.

Detoxify and cleanse the colon through fasting and internal cleansing. Never overwork and overuse the colon; in other words, eat less, or eat only when hungry.

The front door

The front door includes the urinary system (the kidneys, the uterus, the bladder, and the urethra), as well as the genital system (penis, vagina, ovaries, and testes). The urinary system maintains the levels of water, pH, hormones, and minerals of the body, while the genital system is responsible for sexual and reproduction activities.

Manage the opening of the front door—both the urinary system and the genital system—with the balance and coordination of all body organs associated with digestion, absorption, and elimination of the digestive system.

All in all, take conscious care of all the nine openings to slow down your health degeneration.

If you just don't die

If you just don't die, there will be many more changes in your life. You just have to adapt yourself to the changes, or simply have to change yourself accordingly.

Life Challenges

Changes may ultimately become challenges when they are increasingly intense and inevitable. Life challenges may come in different forms.

Physical loss

Physical loss includes loss of vision and mobility, both of which may ultimately affect the quality of life with respect to independent living. Physical loss may also include the loss of limbs due to accidents or disease, such as diabetes.

Material loss

Material loss may include loss of place and space, such as moving from a house to an apartment, or to a nursing home. Downsizing also means the loss or forced disposal of treasured possessions.

Just learn to let go of your attachments. Dispose of or give away some of your belongings and possessions, that is, to de-clutter your living environment as early as possible. Don't procrastinate; do it *now* while you still have the organizational ability and the physical strength to go through your possessions to retrieve what are the most important to you. Don't leave the burden to others, especially your loved ones, such as your children and grandchildren!

Mental loss

Memory loss may result in a severe loss of organizational ability and the ability to plan and function, resulting in loss of independence, which is a major setback for many. Mental loss may also result from the devastating Alzheimer's disease

Spousal loss

Spousal loss is often the most devastating in that the oneness in marriage is forever broken. Anyway, inevitable as it is, learn to be independent and self-sufficient to mitigate the intensity of spousal loss, which may come at some point in your life.

Spiritual loss

Spiritual loss is the loss of meaning and purpose in life, which can lead to a rapid decline in health or even death. Near the end of one's life journey, the will to live is contingent on having a meaning and a purpose to live for.

Hope is a positive meaning to live for. In addition, to love and to be loved may give you joy, without which life has little meaning. Even an infant needs to be loved, cuddled, and hugged in order to remain healthy, physically, mentally, and spiritually. Everyone needs to love and be loved, especially those in their senior years. Family connection, through e-mails, letters, and phone calls, provides a purpose to keep on keeping on. Continue to make new friends and expand your social circle at any stage in your life.

Trust is essential to living a meaningful and purposeful life. Unfortunately, many seniors develop suspicion, distrust, and even paranoia. Don't give up trusting others; don't cut off your lifeline to others who supply your basic needs; don't isolate yourself with cynicism and suspicion that close the door to healthy relationships. Always give people the benefit of the doubt. Always think positive about others around you!

Death and dying

Death is the end of one's life journey.

Have you ever wondered why humans have to become frail and fragile at the end? Maybe it is the Creator's purpose to make them let go of everything on this earth in order to prepare them for their last journey to Him.

On the final journey, with acceptance of the inevitable fate, there is usually no anger or depression—just numbness that initiates the winding down of the body.

Dying is just something we all have to do. Do you want to die with grace? Dying with grace is to end well. All is well that ends well!.

Francis of Assisi, the Italian saint who chose a life of poverty in spite of his family's wealth, said on his deathbed: "Death will open the door of life." He died gracefully while singing.

Maybe for a believer, death is, indeed, a triumph, a meaningful exodus from this mundane world. For a non-believer, death is just the end of everything, and that is what life is all about.

If you just don't die

If you just don't die, you just have to accept and embrace all your life challenges, especially when you cannot change them, nor can you change yourself.

> And the LORD, He *is* the One who goes before you. He will be with you, He will not leave you nor forsake you; do not fear nor be dismayed."
> (**Deuteronomy** 31:8)

> "Understanding the comings and goings of things,
> we fret not, and judge not.
> Focusing on the Creator,
> we are open to all of life.
> Opening to all of life,
> we embrace all with thankfulness for what we get,
> with gratitude for not getting what we deserve.
> Discovering the true nature of things,
> we live with compassion and loving-kindness.
> All endings become beginnings, all returning to the Creator."
> (Lao Tzu, *Tao Te Ching*, chapter 16)

SEVEN

CONSCIOUSNESS OF BEING

"To be yourself in a world that is constantly trying to make you something else is the greatest accomplishment." **Ralph W. Emerson**

In order to live your life as if everything is a miracle, you must change, as well as accept and embrace any challenge in your life. Don't shrink back from the challenge of change. Don't expect others around you to change in order to let you get what you want in your life. If your body, mind, and soul are in total harmony with one another, everything in your life will naturally fall into its right place. Then, no matter at what stage in your life, you will see all possibilities of reaching your dreams, and you will see no void between what you already have and what you want.

Believing in Yourself

Maybe now you are pushing 60, or maybe you have

already crossed the 65-year landmark and beyond. Wherever you may be at this point in time, believe in yourself.

After going through decades of harsh realities in life, you might have become one of those people who find their lives "too harsh" and "too real" to accept; if that is the case, you may now need a good dose of "fantasies" in order to make them more acceptable and ameliorable to you—just like living in your second childhood, and starting to believe in just about anything.

Believing in yourself is like believing in God; it may require what the famous English poet **Coleridge** called "suspension of disbelief." Believe the unthinkable! Just like believing in God, what do you have to lose in believing the unbelievable? In life, there are many things that are no more than thoughts of wishful thinking, just like children believing that Santa Claus would bring them presents if they behave themselves. We all have to believe in *something* in order to make some sense out of our otherwise seemingly senseless existence. If you don't believe in God, at least believe in yourself.

Believing in yourself was one of the first steps to success in anything you achieved when you were young in years. Remember, how you began your first steps when you were a toddler—you *believed* you could walk, and you *did*. Believing in yourself is one of the most important first steps to happiness, especially if you are already advanced in years.

It is important that you believe in yourself—believing that you *can* do what you have to do; believing that you can *still* make waves in the final chapters of your life. In every endeavor in life, beginning the journey is as important as reaching its destination. Make your way through your life journey by doing what needs to be done, and by believing that you *can* do it no matter how and no matter what! Begin your journey of self-belief.

Living is about *doing*. If you do not do what you can do, and do not do what you have to do, you are essentially not living. Believing in yourself provides you not only with a compass but also a roadmap so that you can finish your life journey and reach your final destination. Do what you want to do, and turn your dreams into realities. Just start believing in yourself!

Obstacles to believing in yourself

Believing in yourself, however, is not always that easy, especially as you continue to age. There are two obstacles that you must first overcome before you can start believing in yourself *again*.

The obstacle of comparing

Do not compare yourself with others, or even with your own past, such as your health or past achievements. It is not uncommon that at some point in your life you would compare yourself with others only to observe where you are or how you are doing. However, by comparing too much and too often—especially in your advanced years—you may end up judging yourself as well as others. Comparing and judging do not help you in believing in yourself.

There was an ancient Chinese fable of a stonecutter who worked so hard cutting stones that he often felt stressed and depressed.

One day, while standing behind a huge stone where he was cutting his stones, he looked up at the sky, and saw the beautiful sun. Then, he wished he were the sun that could give warmth and sunshine to everyone on earth. A fairy came to him and granted him his wish, so he became the sun.

For a while, he was happy and contented. Then, one day, a big cloud came over, blocked out everything from his view, and he could not even see what was below and beyond. He became distressed, and wished he were the cloud, instead of the sun. Again, the fairy came to his rescue, and granted him his wish. He became the cloud, and began drifting and floating happily and peacefully in the sky.

After a while, a strong wind came and scattered the cloud in different directions. Now, he wished he were the strong wind that could blow away anything and everything that stood in his way. Again, the fairy made his wish come true: he became the strong wind, blowing here and there. For a while, he was happy and contented.

Then, one day, he found out that he could not blow away the big stone behind which he used to cut stones. Worse, he was stuck there, going nowhere. Now, finally, he realized that was where he belonged. He made his one last wish to become the stonecutter that he used to be. The fairy granted him his last wish, and now he was contented to be the stonecutter again.

The moral of the fable: comparison and contrast between yourself and others is often a stumbling block to self-contentment, without which there is no self-discovery, which is the ultimate enlightenment of believing in yourself.

The obstacle of looking back

Any comparison at any stage in life may lead to guilt and regret. It is pointless to lament or regret over what you had done or should not have done. Don't look back in anger or with bitterness, remorse, or disappointment. The past was all gone and irretrievable. Make peace with your past. Don't yearn over what was or what might have been! Don't dwell on what you have lost! Only look *forward* to the days ahead, and do whatever you have set your mind to do! Just learn to come to terms with what you have. Now is as good a time as any to begin a new chapter, be it the last one in your life, and make it a good and memorable one at that!

Believing in Others

The poet **John Donne** once said: "No man is an island." That is to say, we are all somehow and somewhat inter-connected with one another. This universal moral principle may lead you to true freedom and profound wisdom in living. Once you understand that the life flowing in your veins is the same as that flowing in the veins of others, you may then learn *how* to show your love and compassion towards others. After all, we are *all* created in the image of the Creator, and, therefore, we are no more and no less than the expressions of His creation.

The consciousness of the oneness of all life may also deliver you from the bondage of anger, competitiveness, disrespect, discrimination, envy, hatred, ridicule, and many other negative attitudes and toxic thoughts that might have been stored in your mind, and thus adversely affecting your thinking, which controls your life.

The oneness of all life may further make you realize that you are not much different from others, and that all have different or similar imperfections. That notion may make it easier for you not only to accept yourself as who you are, as well as others as who they are, but also to love them just as you love yourself. Love and compassion are expressions of the oneness of all life—a mental attitude that liberates human bondage from the ego-self, which often focuses on distinguishing and separating the self from others.

Believing in yourself is critical to loving yourself and

loving others. This *connectedness* may help you believe in others, which is essentially trust, a byproduct of love. Trust is an essential element in living a meaningful and purposeful life. Unfortunately, many people develop suspicion, distrust, and even paranoia, especially as they continue to age. Learning to trust is one of life's most difficult tasks. Do not give up trusting others; do not cut off your lifeline to others; do not isolate yourself with cynicism and suspicion that close the door to healthy relationships. Always give people the benefit of the doubt. Think positive about others around you!

Just remember that every person has a heart, and every heart has a place to love and to be loved, as well as to be connected to other hearts. Avail yourself of every opportunity in life to express your love and care to others. You pass through life only once, so show your compassion and loving-kindness *now*, and not later.

There was a Jewish story of a man who died and was shown two images in both heaven and hell, in which people were sitting at both sides of a long table with a meal before each of them. He noticed that the people in hell were starving, because each of them had a spoon that was much too long to fit into his or her own mouth. However, the people in heaven were well fed, because each was using the same long spoon to feed the person *across* the table.

Believing in Spirituality

Love and compassion, generosity and gratitude, sympathy and empathy—they are the stepping stones to believing in spirituality.

We are now living in a secular society, where science is the dominant religion. As a result, many people do not believe in the existence of God. Despite the absence of God in their lives, spirituality may still be present in the hearts of many because they still believe that they have a soul, which is essentially an unfathomable spirit that provides the mind of an individual with direction, guidance, and understanding.

For those who believe in God, the soul is the *connection* to God. This connection is a line of spiritual communication in the form of prayers, moments of self-awakening, and divine inspiration.

For those who do not have a specific religion, but still believe in the control of a Being greater than themselves, the spirit is the deep *understanding* of the inexplicable control and the natural cycle of things—certain things in life that are beyond human control and understanding; certain things in life that follow a natural cycle or order, such as life is inevitably followed by death.

For those who are non-believers, but decent human beings, the spirit is the *conscience* that can tell them what is right and wrong, and not just following the law and order.

Therefore, in different ways, we all have a spirit of some sort, although some of us may separate ourselves from it, either consciously or unconsciously. The spirit is like a shadow of ourselves: sometimes we see more of it, and sometimes we see less of it, but It is always within us, part and parcel of our being, forever following us wherever we go, whether we like it or not.

Becoming and transformation

Believing in spirituality may give you the miracle of becoming and transformation.

At some point in your life, especially as you continue to age, you may begin to sense your incompleteness, your loneliness, your limitations, your disillusion with human vanity, and you may begin to long for someone or something that can truly fill and satisfy you or your inner longing. In your youth, you might have turned to the physical world to gratify your needs and wants, such as successful careers, material comforts, and satisfying relationships, among others. At some point in your life, however, you may sudden realize that your past wayward pursuits were in vain—much like "chasing after the wind" (**Ecclesiastes** 2, 11), and that you have deviated from your conscience and distanced yourself from spirituality or your Creator.

Believing in spirituality may enhance your consciousness of your true self with the deep desire to become wholesome. Becoming is a miracle of transformation of your whole being. Change is external, but transformation is internal. Change requires you to look outside of you; transformation comes from looking inside of you.

Eckhart Tolle, the author of *The Power of Now*, says in the beginning of the book:

> "A beggar has been sitting by the side of a road for over thirty years. One day a stranger walked by. 'Spare some change?' mumbled the beggar, mechanically holding out his old baseball cap. 'I have nothing to give you,' said the stranger. Then he asked: 'What's that you are sitting on?' 'Nothing,' replied the beggar. 'Just an old box. I have been sitting on it for as long as I can remember.' 'Ever looked inside?' asked the stranger. 'No,' said the beggar. 'What's the point? There's nothing in there.' 'Have a look inside,' insisted the stranger. The beggar managed to pry open the lid. With astonishment, disbelief, and elation, he saw that the box was filled with gold."

Change may have a negative connotation in that you

want to get rid of something undesirable in order to receive something desirable; while transformation is enhancement of something which in itself is good, and which is already innate in you. Transformation is rediscovery of what is already there, but has somehow become invisible to the naked eye of the body, imperceptible to the mind, and unintelligible to the soul due to their misalignment. Transformation is often the pathway to enlightenment

The miracle of becoming is to help yourself be what you are meant to be—that is, *being* your "real" self. It is not what you want to be, what you wish you were, or what others think you should be. Being is the outcome of your becoming and transformation. With the miracle of being, you have new perceptions of your true self, and you begin to appreciate *who* you are, and *why* you are here. In other words, you begin to feel your own self-worth, which is a gift from your Creator, and you begin to derive your physical and emotional fulfillment from that source.

If You Just Don't Die

Remember, if you just don't die, change is continuous, and transformation is subtle and significant. You have to be conscious of the change that is happening to you and around you. Life is forever kneading you in many different ways. You can choose to derive either joy or suffering from it. There are different ways to take charge of your life: through the body, the mind, and the soul. The choice is yours.

Physically, to take charge of your life through the body may be a little difficult at first, but it is a sure way because you can *see* what works and what does not.

Mentally, it may be more difficult to take charge of your life through the mind because you may *think* you are doing well but the people around you may say otherwise. Your body always tells you the truth, but your mind may lie to you.

Spiritually, the soul is often the most difficult to access because you are living in a physical world with too many material attachments and distractions. Let go to let God take charge of your life.

EIGHT

YOU JUST DON'T DIE

"Life is a song—sing it. Life is a game—play it. Life is a challenge—meet it. Life is a dream—realize it. Life is a sacrifice—offer it. Life is love—enjoy it." **Sai Baba**

What would happen to you, if you just don't die, and you are now in your eighties, nineties, or even 100 and beyond?

Just go on living as if there were no tomorrow.

But what if you are like many who are burdened with memory loss, physical impairment, and sexual inactivity, and who are now left behind with aches and pains, emotionally devastated by loss and bereavement of their loved ones, haunted by their own regrets and frustrations in the past, and plagued by fear and despair of the future ahead?

Just go on with your life as if there were no yesterday, and there is only today.

On the other hand, if you are happy about your golden years, congratulations! Just go on with the notion that death is something that can be denied or even ignored but can never be avoided.

Just remember the following aspects of wisdom:

The Wisdom to Perceive

Feeling about aging is no more than your subjective perception of the self. It is always the "glass is half full or half empty" attitude of looking at life. More specifically, it is how you view your own life "in the eyes of the beholder" who is nobody but *you*.

If you have strong self-efficacy, which is your self-belief, you will retain better control of your life at any phase of your life; you will feel more capable and competent to seek any opportunity to better your life by overcoming any worry and pessimism.

According to a study of the Harvard School of Public Health, Americans are pessimistic about their health. To illustrate, according to the study, 40 percent of Americans believed they would get breast cancer at some point in their lives, but only 10 percent actually got the disease. A case in point, actress **Angelina Jolie** had her breasts removed out of her belief in the reality of becoming yet another breast cancer victim.

Negative stereotypes

To change any negative subjective perception of aging, you must remove all negative stereotypes associated with aging or the elderly. Aging is not a disease, neither is it only despair and disability. You should not view aging as a personality homogenizer, that is, at some point in time, like everybody else, you will lose your own individuality and fall into a common category known as the elderly, or the senile and the decrepit.

Myths and truths

The myth: you inevitably feel much older as you advance in years.

The truth: quite the contrary, according to a 2009 Pew Research survey, many seniors feel that they are 10 to19 years younger, not older, than their chronological age.

The myth: dementia is inevitable in life.

The truth: dementia is only one of the many symptoms of Alzheimer's disease. If you don't have the disease, you may only have some senior moments, which are just momentary memory lapses. Use it or lose it. If you regularly use and exercise your brain, you will have fewer senior moments. Of course, if you do have the Alzheimer's disease, then it is something else.

The myth: you can no longer exercise your body and mind in your 50s, 60s, and beyond.

The truth: you can always exercise, despite your aches and pains. As a matter of fact, immobility aggravates muscle weakness and inflexibility, and thus creating a vicious circle of inactivity and pain.

The myth: you are too old to give up your nicotine.

The truth: research studies have indicated that most seniors are able to give up their lifelong habit of smoking. If you are a smoker, you can still give up your addiction, if you choose to.

The myth: you can never teach an old dog new tricks.

The truth: scientists have found that the cognitive reserve in the human brain enables learning new things in the latter half of life. Whether you wish to continue to empower yourself with new knowledge in your senior years is your personal choice, and it has little to do with your mind power or your age.

The myth: elderly women are more likely to develop depression than men.

The truth: according to National Women's Health Resources, elderly women often become more adventurous and more ready to look for new opportunities in life than men do.

The myth: depression is a disease that will impair an aging body and mind.

The truth: depression is a treatable medical condition. Just don't stigmatize yourself!

The Wisdom to Understand

Adversity

Adversity is part and parcel of life and living. Adversity coming in different phases only becomes more challenging and noticeable in your advanced years. Therefore, it is important to understand the nature of adversity in order to cope with it, not necessarily to overcome it.

Adversity is like the rites of passage, which come in three stages: the separation stage in which you feel separated from your comfort zone; the confusion stage in which you find yourself in no-man's-land, at a complete loss of not knowing what to do next; and the transformation stage, in which you initiate the changes to cope with the adversity.

Pain

Pain comes in different forms: emotional, physical, mental, and spiritual pain. Inevitable as it is, pain also comes in different stages of life, and most predominantly during the last years as a result of loss of loved ones, loss of physical capability and functioning, as well as loss of health and wellness.

According to **Dr. Albert Schweitzer,** "'Pain is a more terrible lord of mankind than even death itself, and awakens us to a courage and faith unrealized before."

No matter what, your last years will ultimately dwindle into your days of peace and harmony—what is experienced by those who accept and embrace pain. Humor and laughter are the only antidotes to pain.

Norman Cousins, in his book *Anatomy of an Illness*, was able to cure himself of terminal cancer by exposing himself to as much humor as he could get from movies and comic books. No matter what, smile, laugh, and develop a sense of humor.

Smiling

Babies begin smiling within the first few weeks of life, and laugh out loud within months of being born because laughter is a natural, positive response to human life. Sadly, as human life progresses, laughter begins to fade away into oblivion.

But laughter is especially important to you in the last chapters of your life because it overcomes adversities and all bad feelings about yourself, others, or what is happening to you. Laughter is your best medicine in your last days: it releases endorphins to make you feel good about yourself no matter what; it protects your heart by improving blood flow to your heart; it reduces your stress hormones, thereby boosting your immune system; it relaxes your body and mind to enable you to enjoy living in the present; it makes you forget your lingering physical and emotional pain. Laughter is your natural medicine for you as you approach the final destination of your life journey.

Humor

While laughter is instantaneous, humor is subtle, gradual, but infectious. The major role of humor in life is to change your perspective of what is happening to you. It enables you to look at yourself in a less serious manner. Since you are dying anyway, why should you look upon life so seriously? Weave humor into the fabrics of your life: let yourself find good humor in everything you do. Remind yourself that you are much more blessed than most people (for one thing, you already have lived to a ripe old age) and that many things are beyond your control anyway, so loosen up your tight jaw and start smiling. Laugh at yourself by sharing some embarrassing moments in your life with those who are fun and playful. Look for humor in any bad situation; if you look further, you will always find the irony and absurdity of life. Above all, make a conscious effort to overcome your daily stress, which is a major impediment to laughter and humor.

According to the 2006 *International Journal of Psychiatry in Medicine*, a sense of humor can significantly improve the survival rate of end-stage renal disease patients by as much as 30 percent. The reason is simple: positive distractions from stressful situations, such as dialysis, have salutary effects on the patient.

Remember, if you just don't die, you will continue to face many challenges and problems. Laughter and humor will let you see their positive sides, instead of becoming the problems yourself.

You do not have to be funny in order to have a sense of humor—just the ability to see the lighter side of life. Now that you are nearing the end of your life journey, nothing can be that dead serious—not even death.

Developing a sense of humor

Developing your sense of humor requires a different perspective on things in life. Changing your perspective means going back through your entire life and looking at all the belief systems that you have inculcated through different experiences in different stages of your life. It is not as simple as you may think, but it is worth the effort, because a good sense of humor may help you in your adversity. Life is full of problems, especially in the last golden days. A good sense of humor controls how you *see* your problems in your daily life.

There are several ways to develop a good sense of humor:

Always see yourself not in the center of things, but rather a part of it. Your problems may not be uniquely yours; others may have the same problems, and, even worse than yours, for that matter. Don't be too self-centered that you are always bearing the blunt.

Never take yourself too seriously. Just learn to laugh at yourself—your mistakes, your foolishness, and even your weaknesses. Remember, nobody is perfect!

Live in the present. Everything is constantly changing, including your body and thoughts. Everything in life can only be experienced in each moment, and moment by moment, which is the only reality. Live in the present moment, appreciate it, and enjoy it to the fullest. When you do just that, you may see not only the humor but also the absurdity of everything around you.

Always putting a smile on your face not only helps you develop a sense of humor but also gives joy to others.

Remember, a smile is contagious. There is no harm in smiling—even in a bad situation.

Make a list of all the things you enjoy in life—things that really make you happy. Remember and recall them at all times.

If you can *laugh* at yourself and join in with the laughter of others, it can bring not only much more joy but also many more golden days to your life.

Final Words of Wisdom

Life might not have been fair to you with happenings that might have been beyond your control. No matter what, life is not meant to be a punishment for you. If you just don't die, you will have the wisdom to live it through.

> "Life begets death; one is inseparable from the other.
>
> One is form; the other is formless.
>
> Each gives way to the other.
> One third of people focus on life, ignoring death.
> One third of people focus on death, ignoring life.
> One third of people think of neither, just drifting along.
> They all suffer in the end.
>
> Trusting the Creator, we have no illusion about life and death.
> Holding nothing back from life, we are ready for death,
> just as a man ready for sleep after a good day's work."

(Lao Tzu, *Tao Te Ching*, chapter 50)

"Abiding in the Creator, we do not fear death.
Following the conditioned mind, we fear everything.
Fear is a futile attempt to control things and people.

Death is a natural destination of the Way.
Unnatural fear of death does more harm than good.
It is like trying to use intricate tools of a master craftsman:
we end up hurting ourselves."
(Lao Tzu, *Tao Te Ching*, chapter 74)

If you just don't die, the wisdom in living the rest of your life is no more than . . .

Just like eating a meal

Living the rest of your life is just like eating a meal.

Before your start your meal, say your grace. (Just like being grateful and thankful that you just don't die and that you can still have this meal.)

Before you pick up your food, take a minute or two to still your mind. There is no need to hurry; you've all the time in the world to finish this meal. (Just like being conscious of living in the now.)

There is no right or wrong about eating the food in front of you—eating is just a process, a way of living and surviving, just like breathing in and out. (Just like knowing that now you don't need to eat to socialize, to relieve stress, to satisfy your food cravings, or to make yourself feel better—you eat simply because you just don't die.)

Look at the food in front of you. Notice the color, the smell, and the texture of the food. (Just like being conscious of the people and the happenings around you.)

Now, begin eating. No matter how small the bite of food you have, take at least two bites. Take your first bite. Chew it *very* slowly but thoroughly, noticing and enjoying your actual sensory experience of chewing and tasting. Chew every morsel of food to explore the differences in their taste, texture, and smell. (Just like enjoying whatever that is still available to you that you still find enjoyable.)

Continue to eat in silence without any distraction. (Just like you continue to live without being distracted by what might happen tomorrow.)

Just like watching a suspense movie

Living in the last days is also like watching a suspense movie, full of unpredictable twists and turns: you don't know *how* it would end until the very end; otherwise, it wouldn't be worth watching. Don't turn your head away, and don't cover your eyes with your hands. Just watch and *enjoy* the movie!

APPENDIX A

THE WISDOM OF LIVING TO 100 AND BEYOND

If you just don't die, living to 100 and beyond may not be an impossibility if you just follow some basic recipes for longevity living.

The Art of Eating

You eat to live, and not live to eat; your food is always your medicine. Eat only when you are hungry; never eat to satisfy your cravings.

The best foods

According to **Dr. Mao Shing Ni**, the natural-health expert on Yahoo, the ten top best foods are:

1. Sweet potatoes
2. Corn
3. Peanuts
4. Pumpkin

5. Walnuts
6. Black beans
7. Sesame seeds
8. Shiitake mushrooms
9. Green tea
10. Seaweed

Of course, there are many other healthy foods that should also be included in any healthy diet.

Healthy fruits

Apple: brain and immunity health
Avocado: healthy cholesterol
Banana: fat burning
Cantaloupe: anti-inflammation, and immunity health
Kiwi: bowel health
Mango: artery health
Orange: cholesterol health
Papaya: fat burning
Pineapple: asthma
Plum and prune: bowel health
Watermelon: fertility, and skin health

Healthy berries

Blackberries: fat burning, bone health
Blueberries: brain health
Cherries: anti-inflammation
Cranberries: prostate health
Raspberries: cholesterol health
Strawberries: anti-inflammation, and brain health

Healthy vegetables

Artichoke: cholesterol health
Asparagus: heart health
Broccoli: brain health
Butternut squash: heart health
Carrot: vision health
Cauliflower: prostate health
Cabbage: detoxification
Kale: bone health
Pumpkin: anti-inflammation, and cholesterol health
Red bell pepper: heart health
Spinach: mental health and sharpness
Sweet potato: vision health
Tomato: anti-inflammation, and heart health

The food types

Okinawa in Japan has more centenarians than the rest of the world. The diet of Okinawa centenarians, for example, derives 85% of calories from carbohydrate, 9% from protein, and 6% from fat.

The food digestion

Digestion is an important aspect of eating. Your food must be digested within three hours. Food not digested within three hours has two implications: the wrong kind of food, or the wrong quantity of food for your body.

When it comes to food, one of the most important aspects that you must be conscious of is how quickly a certain type of food is digested and becomes a part of yourself. If the food moves out of your stomach within three hours, it means that even if it is not the best food, it is still something your system is able to handle.

If you maintain a clear gap of five to six hours between meals, internal cleansing will happen on the cellular level. This cleansing on the cellular level is most important for a healthful life. If you are a senior, two good meals a day will suffice—one in the morning and one in the early evening.

There must be three hours after the evening meal, before you go to bed. This should also include at least 20 to 30 minutes of light physical activity, such as simple walking, to ensure a healthy digestive system.

The Miracle of Doing

When it comes to doing, one simple thing that you need to remember is that your body is capable of bending forward, bending backward, twisting to both sides. and squatting. This miracle of doing must happen in some kind of form as a part of your daily life so that your spinal column is stretched. This miracle of doing is a must if you want to keep your entire body system healthy—especially your neurological system, which will otherwise be an issue as you continue to age.

The Power of Thoughts

Humans have a mental body. The mind is not in one particular part of the body; as a matter of fact, every cell in the human body has its own memory and intelligence. This mental body is also responsible for human thoughts. The physical body is the hardware; the mental body is the software. Take good care of both the hardware and the software to optimize the functioning of your computer.

The Benefits of Rituals

Rituals have many benefits, including the subliminal

suggestion of continuity.

Bedtime rituals

You spend at least one third of your time staying in bed. Have you ever thought of doing some bedtime rituals? They are conducive to your longevity as well as beneficial to your health and well-being. Any daily ritual suggests continuity.

Before going to bed or while lying on your bed, do the following:

- Lie on your back. Bend both knees.
- Use both hands to pull your knees towards your chest, and breathe naturally.
- Hold for one to two minutes, and relax.
- Straighten your legs, putting your arms and hands at your sides. Relax for one to two minutes.
- Now, take a deep breath, and stretch both arms upwards above your head.
- Then, slowly bring your hands down while you breathe out.
- Massage your body from your chest to your abdomen for a few minutes.
- Bring both hands at your sides, and relax.
- Repeat as necessary until you feel drowsy and fall asleep.

Morning rituals

Research studies have shown that most heart attacks occur in the morning due to the sudden changes from sleep to wakefulness.

Follow the ancient Chinese Taoist monks' rituals of

waking up to have a clear mind and a healthy body:

- Use your fingertips to massage your ears, eyes, lips, and nose.
- Gently tap your scalp with your hands.
- With a continual stroking action, massage your shoulders, elbows, hands, chest, abdomen, knees, and feet.
- With your palms, massage your lower back.
- Then inhale vigorously through your nose, and exhale forcefully through your mouth several times in order to rid your body of toxins.

In addition, do some "wake-up" stretches before you get up to "awaken" body and your senses, thereby instrumental in preventing aches and pains in your body. **Dr. Robert Oexman**, director of the Sleep to Live Institute, also stressed the importance of stretching your back before getting up: "The greatest incidence of slipped discs occurs within 30 to 60 minutes after we wake up."

- Extend your arms over your head and extend your legs as far as possible, as evidenced by the stretch in the tips of your fingers and toes.
- Meanwhile, inhale deeply through your nose.
- Then breathe out deeply and slowly while drawing your arms down along the side your body with your palms facing up. You will feel full relaxation in your legs. Repeat the stretches several times to energize as well as to relax your body.

In addition, do a single or double knee hug.

- Bring your knee into your chest.
- Massage your hip joint by moving your leg in circles in both directions.
- Repeat with the other knee.
- Finally, hug both knees into your chest, raising your nose to your knees as much as possible.
- Now relax your body and let your knees fall gently down to either side.
- Repeat the whole process several times for stretch and relaxation.

As soon as you get out of bed, practice the ritual of making your own saliva, which is your body's own built-in self-made fluid for self-defense against viruses and infections. Harness the power of this miracle fluid to make your own saliva as much as possible.

- On waking up each morning, stand erect.
- Gently exhale through the mouth three times to rid your body of toxins accumulated during your sleep.
- Close your mouth, and begin hitting your teeth for 30 seconds as if you were chewing food in your mouth.
- Then, slowly massage your teeth with your tongue for 30 seconds.
- By then, your mouth should have generated some saliva. Do not swallow it immediately. Instead, close your eyes, and visualize that your are swallowing the saliva, and it is slowly dripping down to the *dan tian*, the "energy center" of your body, which is located in the lower abdomen between the navel and the pubic bone. The *dan*

tian is also a source of power for physical energy, sexual vitality, and inner power as emphasized by the Chinese Qi Gong exercise.

- Now, slowly swallow your saliva.

According to Eastern medicine, human saliva has miraculous healing power. Research in a recent Japanese study indicated that saliva can even fight cancer cells in rats and other animals.

For thousands of years, Chinese physicians have believed that saliva has all the ingredients for longevity and overall wellness due to its inherent benefits on the five human organs: the heart, liver, spleen, lungs, and kidneys. Saliva is anti-aging because it promotes cell growth and cell division.

For natural oral health, clean your mouth with sesame oil.

- To remove a film of impurities from your tongue, gargle a tablespoonful of warm sesame oil for a minute or two; spit out the oil.
- Use a tongue scraper to scrape your tongue until all the white coating is gone.
- Gently massage your gums with your fingers.

Use warm sesame oil for oral hygiene, instead of the harsh commercial mouthwash. Sesame oil helps you purify your colon as well as improve your digestion. Sesame oil is especially good for removing harmful bacteria from your mouth and preventing gum disease. Research studies have shown that swishing and gargling sesame oil is best for gum disease and cavity for better oral health. In addition, sesame oil has the benefits of strengthening your jaws, preventing cracked lips and sore throat.

APPENDIX B

THE WISDOM OF CENTENARIANS

The Ancient Centenarian: Luigi Cornaro

Luigi Cornaro, a Venetian nobleman, was one of the most celebrated centenarians, who lived from 1464 to 1566 AD.

In his youth, Luigi had abused his health with a lifestyle of wantonness and excess, resulting in an extremely weak constitution, accompanied by many physical ailments.

At the age of thirty-five, he was given up by his physicians to die. Luigi's physicians prescribed a temperate lifestyle as the only way to end his suffering and preserve his very fragile life. That temperate lifestyle was essentially the exercise of self-restraint or self-discipline in relation to diet and drink for calorie restriction. His physician recommended for him a diet consisting of only twelve ounces a day of solid foods of bread, a vegetable soup with tomato, an egg yolk, and a little meat, divided into two meals, and fourteen ounces of pure grape juice, also divided into two servings.

He lived on that minimal diet of calorie restriction from age thirty-five until eighty-five, when his relatives began to urge him to eat a little more since he was getting old and he required more physical strength and stamina. Complying with and succumbing to their well wishes and importunities, Luigi reluctantly agreed to increase his food intake from twelve to fourteen ounces. Immediately, he became seriously ill with high fever. Eventually, Luigi had the longevity wisdom to revert to his former anti-aging living with a diet of calorie restriction. As a result, he lived in a state of unbroken health and happiness until the age of one hundred and two.

Luigi was famous for his longevity living in relation to calorie restriction. He expressed his wisdom in his discourse when he was in his eighties and nineties. His wisdom has been an inspiration for more than five centuries. His longevity wisdom was simple and down-to-earth: never overeat; avoid environmental stress, such as extreme heat and cold; and avoid extreme fatigue, and interruption of sleep.

The bottom line: you don't have to eat such a low-calorie diet of Luigi in order to live long; just eat *less*, and eat only when you are hungry.

The Contemporary Centenarian: Dr. Shigeaki Hinohara

Dr. Shigeaki Hinohara, from Japan, turned 104 recently, and he is one of the world's longest-serving physicians and educators. Since 1941, he has been healing patients at St. Luke's International Hospital in Tokyo and teaching at St. Luke's College of Nursing. He has published around 15 books since his 75th birthday, including his bestseller "Living Long, Living Good."

As the founder of the New Elderly Movement, Hinohara

encourages others to live a long and happy life with the following wisdom he would like to share with all:

- Dr. Shigeaki Hinohara stresses the importance of not becoming overweight.
- For breakfast, Dr. Shigeaki Hinohara drinks coffee, milk, and orange juice with a tablespoon of olive oil, which is for healthy arteries and healthy skin. For lunch, he drinks milk with a few cookies. For dinner, he eats vegetables, a bit of fish and rice, and, sometimes some lean meat.
- He always keeps himelf busy with a full schedule ahead. He recommends that any retirement should be a lot later than 65.
- He shares what he knows—one of the reasons why he is still working and teaching. When he teaches, he always stands to stay strong.
- He recommends having a second thought or always seeking a second opinion whenever a doctor recommends a test, a procedure, or a surgery.
- He believes that doctors cannot cure everyone. Instead, he believes in music and animal therapy.
- He recommends taking the stairs and carrying your own stuff to stay healthier and younger for longer.
- He uses doing fun things to forget his pain, both physical and emotional.
- He recommends letting go of all material things because nobody knows when his or her number is up, and nothing can be taken to the next place.
- He believes that each person is unique, and illness is therefore individualized. But medical

science lumps all and sundry together; an individual should understand why he or she is sick, and not the doctor. Science alone cannot cure or help you; you must learn to help yourself.

- He believes that life is always filled with unpredictable incidents. So, be prepared.
- He stresses the importance of finding a role model to help with setting life goals and life purposes.
- He believes that energy comes from doing good and feeling good, and not from good food or good sleep.
- To Dr. Shigeaki Hinohara, it is always wonderful to live long, and he loves every minute of it.

YOU JUST DON'T DIE!

APPENDIX C

THE MIRACLE OF MEDITATION

Meditation is thinking about one thing at a time. Simple as it may seem, this requires practice and discipline. According to **St. Theresa of Avila**, the mind is like an unbridled horse wandering where it will, and your role is to train the horse, and gently and lovingly bring it back to the right course.

Meditation is training your mental attention to sharpen your consciousness of what is going on in your mind. Once you see clearly what is going on in the present moment, you can then choose to ignore or to act upon what you are seeing through your mind.

For thousands of years, people have been transforming their minds through this simple mind training. Meditation can be done in silence and stillness, through sounds, or even body movements—as long as the focal point is mental attention and awareness of the present moment.

Whatever that gets your attention will control and dominate you. In other words, your habitual responses pre-condition your mind. Therefore, the primary purpose of meditation is to refocus and pay clear attention to your experiences and responses as they go through your mind; you just observe, without judging them. The objective of observing without any judgment is to eliminate as much as possible any automatic and reflexive response that leads to the pre-conditioning of the mind. Simply put, don't jump to conclusion yet; get all the details first, and then evaluate them objectively.

The Meditation Process

Meditation is a simple process that can be practiced by every one of us. The meditation process involves:

- Quieting the mind: observing thoughts and feelings with no judgment
- Controlling the mind: taming a wandering or an overactive mind

The meditation process can last from 10 minutes or so to more than an hour. Just let it happen naturally.

Meditation Basics

To meditate, you must get into the right frame of mind; that is, you must learn some meditation basics in order to know *how* to meditate effectively:

- You must be in a quiet environment conducive to meditation.
- Your body must be comfortable and still, and very relaxed.
- Your breathing must be right: inhale and exhale softly and slowly, preferably in a rhythm.

- Your mind must be focused, staying in the present moment, as much as possible.
- You must not expect anything to happen during the meditation session. You must always practice with consistency and persistence.

How to Meditate

Find a quiet place where you can remain undisturbed for 10 to 30 minutes. To set the environment for meditation, you may want to have some scent from flowers or incense, or even some soothing music (meditation MP3) to enhance your senses. Of course, you can meditate without them; it is just an option, not a requirement.

Find time to practice meditation. Regularity holds the key to success in meditation. Do not meditate only when you feel like it. Find some quiet time to yourself every day. The ideal time to meditate is before retiring to bed; in that way, your mind can review what has happened during the day—what you have said and done—and let go of everything. After all, meditation is about letting go of the past and future thoughts.

Correct posture is important. Firstly, your body must be erect: this induces correct breathing, which can bring all your internal energies into a state of harmony. Therefore, do not lean back on anything. If you find that your neck is too weak and your spine cannot support your body, then rest your back on a hard surface initially; but the ultimate goal is to sit erect without your back touching anything.

You can sit cross-legged on the floor. Alternatively, you can sit comfortably on a chair (not a sofa), with your thighs at right angles to your spine, your hands on your thighs, your feet resting firmly on the floor, and your shoulders relaxed. In short, just sit "tall" and erect.

Begin meditation with your breathing. Your breathing is

an indicator of your stress level: if you are unduly stressed, your breathing becomes thick and gasping. Breathing right is your conscious control of stress. When you feel stressed, consciously change your breathing pace to undo the stress.

Gently close your eyes, or you can fix your eyes on an object, such as a candle.

As you begin your meditation, you will find that your first thought does not come to your mind right away. When it finally comes, do not dismiss it. Instead, consciously focus on your breathing. That thought will then slowly disappear. After a while, another thought or the same thought may come up to your mind. Again, do not consciously dismiss it; refocus on your breathing. With more practice, you will find that within a 10-minute time frame, fewer and fewer thoughts will crop up in your mind because your mind has stayed in the present moment for a longer period. The fewer thoughts you have, the more relaxed you become.

Then, one day, you suddenly find that you have stepped into a different world with total tranquility and clarity of mind—even though it lasts but a very brief moment. That out-of-the-world sensation is nondescript. Once you have attained that inexplicable and transformative state of mind, you will want to continue practicing meditation everyday. But don't expect that transcendental state will come any time soon; the more you expect it, the longer it will take you to attain that state of mind. Just consistently and patiently practice meditation everyday with no expectation other than relaxing your body and mind.

Meditation is life changing, especially in the golden years. Meditation may change *how* you look at yourself and the golden days ahead of you.

APPENDIX D

BIBLIOGRAPHY

Carper, Jean, *Stop Aging Now!*, HarperCollins Publisher, 1995

Chia, Mantak, and Wei, William, *Cosmic Detox*, Destiny Books, 2011

Dauphinais, Marc, *The Incredible Internet Guide to Diets and Nutrition*, Facts on Demand Press, 2000

Davis, Donn M., *Survival Skills for the Modern Man*, Contemporary Books, 1998

Fast, Julie A and Preston, John, *Take Charge of Bipolar Disorder*, Warner Wellness, 2006

Ginsberg, Gary and Toal, Brian, *What's Toxic, What's Not*, Bentley Books, 2006

Heimlich, Jane, *What Your Doctor Won't Tell You*, Harper Perennial, 1990

Johnson, David, *Feel 30 for the Next 50 Years*, Avon Books, 1998

Lau, Stephen, *As If Everything Is A Miracle*, Amazon, 2014

Lau, Stephen, *The Book of Life and Living*, Amazon 2012

Lau, Stephen, *The Complete Tao Te Ching* in Plain English, Amazon, 2016

Lau, Stephen, *The Wisdom of Letting Go*, Amazon, 2016

Lau, Stephen, *Your Golden Years and Santa Claus*, Amazon, 2013

Logan, Alan, *The Brain Diet*, Cumberland House, 2007

Mao Shing Ni, *Dr. Mao's Secrets of Longevity Cookbook*, Andews McMeel, Publishing LLC, 2012

Markowitz, Dave, *Healing with Source*, Findhorn Press, 2010

McQuillan, Susan, *Food Addiction*, Alpha Books, 2004

O'Connor, Richard, *Rewire*, Plume, 2014

Robbins, John, *Healthy at 100*, Thorndike Windsor Paragon, 2006

Towler, Solala, *Tao Paths Long Life*, Andrews McMeel Publishing

Vanderhaeghe, Lorna R, and Bouic, Patrick J.D.., *The Immune System Cure*, Kensington Books, 1999

Vasey, Christopher, *The Acid-Alkaline Diet for Optimum Health*, Healing Arts Press, 1999

ABOUT STEPHEN LAU

About Stephen Lau:

http://www.stephencmlau.com

Books by Stephen Lau:

http://www.booksbystephenlau.com

Stephen Lau's Related Blogs:

http://reflectionsofstephenlau.blogspot.com
http://www.naturalhealthwisdom.com

Stephen Lau's Related Sites:

http://www.health-and-wisdom-tips.com
http://www.wisdominliving.com

Stephen Lau's Newsletter:

http://www.wellness-wisdom-newsletter.com

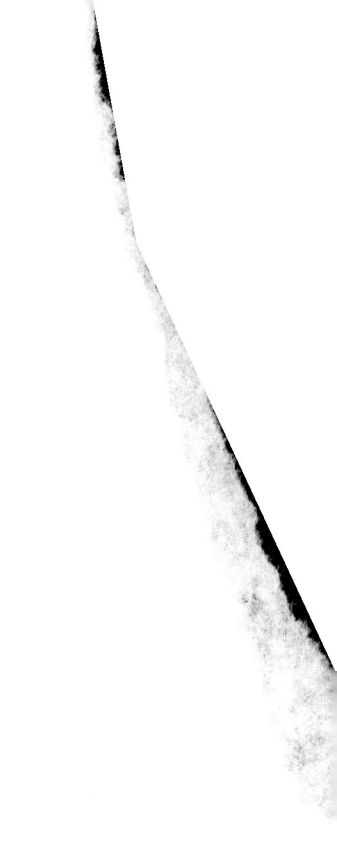

www.ingramcontent.com/pod-product-compliance
Lightning Source LLC
Chambersburg PA
CBHW020518290526
45786CB00002B/653